alli®
Cookbook

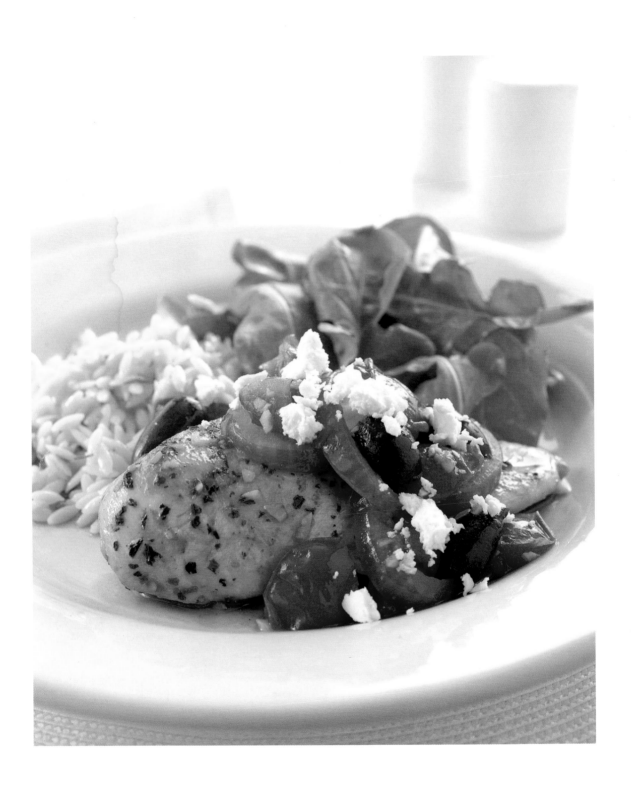

alli®
Cookbook

Chef Contributors

Kathleen Daelemans

Sylvia Meléndez-Klinger

Lindsey Williams

Introduction: Caroline Apovian, M.D.

Produced by The Philip Lief Group, Inc.

Meredith® Books
Des Moines, Iowa

Meredith Books
1716 Locust Street
Des Moines, Iowa 50309-3023
www.meredithbooks.com

First Edition. Printed in the United States of America.
Library of Congress Control Number: 2007925125
ISBN: 978-0-696-23813-0

alli, alli Shuttle, and various design elements are trademarks of GlaxoSmithKline.

READ AND FOLLOW THE LABEL ON
THE alli® PRODUCT BEFORE TAKING.

c o n t e n t s

introduction

Long before I wrote *The alli® Diet Plan*, I was an enthusiastic supporter of orlistat, the active ingredient of alli, not only because the FDA had approved it as safe and effective, but because I witnessed orlistat's positive results firsthand when I prescribed it to my patients. When using alli and moderating your daily fat and calorie intake, you can lose 50 percent more weight than with diet alone. Alli's uniqueness lies in the combination of the efficacy of the capsule and the innovative weight loss program. Together, they help you gradually lose weight.

As a physician nutrition specialist, I have also learned that many people ultimately give up on their diets because of limited or bland food choices and small portions. But you can achieve successful, healthy weight loss without always feeling deprived: You just need to have the right food options. Most important are:

■ Flexibility in the food plan

■ Variety of allowable food

■ Reasonable portion control so you don't feel deprived

■ Good food so you're not tempted to stray

The *alli® Cookbook* brings you just that—a wonderful variety of more than 200 delicious, alli-friendly recipes for breakfast, lunch, dinner, snacks, and desserts that you can mix and match to suit your personal tastes and weight loss goals while keeping fat and calories at the right level.

The recipes in this book are designed to help you lose weight while enjoying some of your favorite classic dishes—such as pancakes, barbecued chicken, clam chowder, and beef tacos. Even dishes you probably thought were forbidden—such as French toast, macaroni and cheese, lasagna, potato casserole, beef stew, and chocolate cake—were specially developed by a team of creative and talented chefs to ensure that you will always have the optimum calorie and fat gram counts while eating great-tasting food. In fact, to maximize the benefits of alli, you can still eat 30 percent of your daily calories from fat, and it's all been precalculated here in these meals. You just have to enjoy. And the portions are generous enough for you to feel satisfied and still lose weight.

Rest assured: This is no boring diet made of micromeals of steamed vegetables. Besides classic dishes, this book provides innovative and international recipes—such as Thai Chicken Chowder, Turkey and Sweet Potato Stew, Marinated Tenderloin in Chipotle Sauce, Gazpacho with Spicy Shrimp, and Curried Chicken Salad Sandwiches. Renowned chef contributors Sylvia Meléndez-Klinger, Lindsey Williams, and Kathleen Daelemans worked with top nutritionists on all the classics and the special recipes for this book, making them alli-friendly while still retaining their great flavors. In fact, these dishes are so tasty you'll even want to make them for friends and family who aren't dieting!

The quick and easy meals in this book along with the extensive resources at *www.myalli.com*

can help you achieve your weight loss goals. At *www.myalli.com* you have access to nutrition and other dieting advice, including an individualized online action plan, dieting tips, and much more with the purchase of alli weight loss capsules. The site also provides you with a supportive online community that will answer questions and help you stay committed to your diet plan.

You've taken an important step by committing yourself to do your best with alli. You have chosen a clinically proven partner to help you gradually lose weight, and *alli Cookbook* will help you achieve your weight loss goals without sacrificing taste. Add this collection of delectable dishes to your recipe repertoire and get cooking—the alli way!

—**Caroline Apovian, M.D.**
Director, Nutrition and Weight Management Center
Codirector, Nutrition and Metabolic Support Service
Boston University Medical Center
Associate Professor of Medicine and Pediatrics
Boston University School of Medicine

eating the alli® way

Losing weight isn't easy, but that doesn't mean that your diet plan has to be complicated. The *alli® Cookbook* makes planning what to eat while you're taking alli weight loss capsules simple—and delicious. Here's how:

If you've purchased this book, you've probably already started to use alli capsules and you are well on your way in your new weight loss plan. Each day you should be consuming approximately 30 percent of your calories from fat and evenly distributing your fat intake over your three main meals. (If you are following *The alli® Diet Plan*, this is Phase 3.) Now you need some more recipes, variety, and flexibility.

Mix and Match

This book offers the flexibility to mix and match meals that are suited to your personal preferences. Conveniently organized by the meals of the day, Breakfast, Lunch, and Dinner, the book also includes three bonus chapters—Little Bites (snacks and appetizers), Desserts, and Holidays—all alli-friendly and all specifically designed to fit into the alli program.

Breakfast, Lunch, and Dinner

In the Breakfast, Lunch, and Dinner chapters, each recipe is either a complete meal or has simple accompaniments provided in order "To Complete the Meal." The nutritional information at the end of each page is for a *Complete Meal Single Serving*, that includes the total fat and calories for the main dish (for which there is a recipe), as well as the side dishes that appear in the "To Complete the Meal" box. So, for example, in the Lemon Roasted Chicken recipe on page 96, the nutritional information reflects a single serving of the Lemon Roasted Chicken in the recipe, and a single serving of the baked potato with sour cream and the broccoli, cauliflower, and peppers

in the "To Complete the Meal" box. All meals are no more than 30 percent calories from fat, so all you have to do is adhere to the portion sizes indicated in the meals, keep track of your daily calorie and fat gram intake, and stay within your personal daily limits. You can choose whichever Breakfast, Lunch, or Dinner meals you like, as long as your total calories and fat grams stay within your target ranges.

for alli® newcomers

If you are just starting your weight loss program with alli weight loss capsules, here's a quick recap of the plan. First you need to determine your daily calorie target—the number of calories you should consume each day based on your gender, current weight, and activity level. You can find your daily calorie target by following the information in the alli Companion Guide or at *www.myalli.com*. Your daily calorie target will then determine how many grams of fat you should consume each day. Remember, you should consume approximately 30 percent of your calories from fat.

On the alli plan is important that you evenly distribute your fat intake throughout the day, both to make a habit of eating a healthy, balanced diet and to eliminate potential treatment effects. For example, if your daily calorie target is 1,800 calories, your daily fat gram total should be 60 grams and you should consume about 20 grams of fat at each meal. Two low-fat snacks that are each 200 calories or less and 3 grams fat or less can also be included. If you are interested in a different option that may help you reduce the chance of treatment effects, you can try the 3-Phase program in *The alli Diet Plan*, by Caroline Apovian, M.D.

Appetizers, Snacks, and Desserts

After a few weeks of getting adjusted to the alli program, you can make your meals even more interesting with the appetizers, snacks, and desserts that are offered. When you add an appetizer or dessert to one of the meals, remember to stay within your calorie and fat target for the meal.

Menu Planning Guidelines

Although many of the Breakfast, Lunch, and Dinner recipes come with complete meal recommendations for side dishes, the appetizers and desserts are up to you to decide. Here are a few easy menu-planning guidelines:

- **Keep track of the calories and fat.** When choosing your appetizer and/or dessert, be sure to add the calories and fat grams to your meal. So, for example, if you decide you want to have Spring Vegetable Lasagna, page 166, for dinner (371 calories / 12 fat g) with a piece of the delicious Flourless Chocolate-Almond Cake, page 226 (103 calories / 3 fat g), your TOTAL calories and fat grams for the meal are 474 calories and 15 fat g. To help you keep track, record your calories and fat grams in the alli Daily Journal that came with your alli starter kit.

- **Don't be confined by chapter titles.** The chapter titles are suggestions for when to enjoy these dishes, but feel free to move meals around to your choosing. So if you'd like to have the Summer Tostada Salad (page 62) from the Lunch chapter for dinner, go right ahead—just be sure to keep your total calories and fat grams within your daily targets.

- **Watch your oil intake.** When taking alli weight loss capsules, too much oil in your food may increase the chance of treatment effects. To help reduce the chance of treatment effects, if the appetizer or dessert that you are adding to a meal contains oil, choose a lunch or dinner menu that is not prepared with oil.

- **"Little Bites" doesn't mean extra bites.** Although some of these appetizer and snack recipes are finger foods, you still must follow the portions allotted for in the recipes. Don't be tempted to sneak in a few extra bites.

- **Don't replace homemade with store-bought.** This book was created to help you enjoy some more healthful versions of traditional favorite foods that might typically be excluded from a weight loss diet. Keep in mind that these recipes have been specifically designed for healthy eating with alli weight loss capsules. So although there may be Buffalo Macaroni and Cheese (page 167) in this book, don't substitute this recipe with store-bought macaroni and cheese—you'll be in for a lot of extra calories and, very likely, too much fat.

Holidays

The holidays are a special time, but they are typically a very difficult time to stay on track with weight loss. The Holidays chapter offers you five alli-friendly menus for special occasions throughout the year. Appetizers, main dishes, side dishes, and desserts are provided to make complete and delicious holiday menus that you don't have to feel guilty about. And your family will love them too.

Easy alli Meal Plans

For weekly meal-planning guidance, the Easy alli Meal Plans chapter provides you with 21 daily menus including breakfast, lunch, dinner, and snacks. The daily menus are offered for each of the four calorie targets: 1,200, 1,400, 1,600, and 1,800 calories. The easy-to-follow daily plans offer a healthy, balanced diet for each of the calorie targets.

Eating the alli way means making smart food choices, exercising moderation and portion control, and balancing your daily fat intake. The *alli* Cookbook helps you do all that without sacrificing taste—or your weight loss goals.

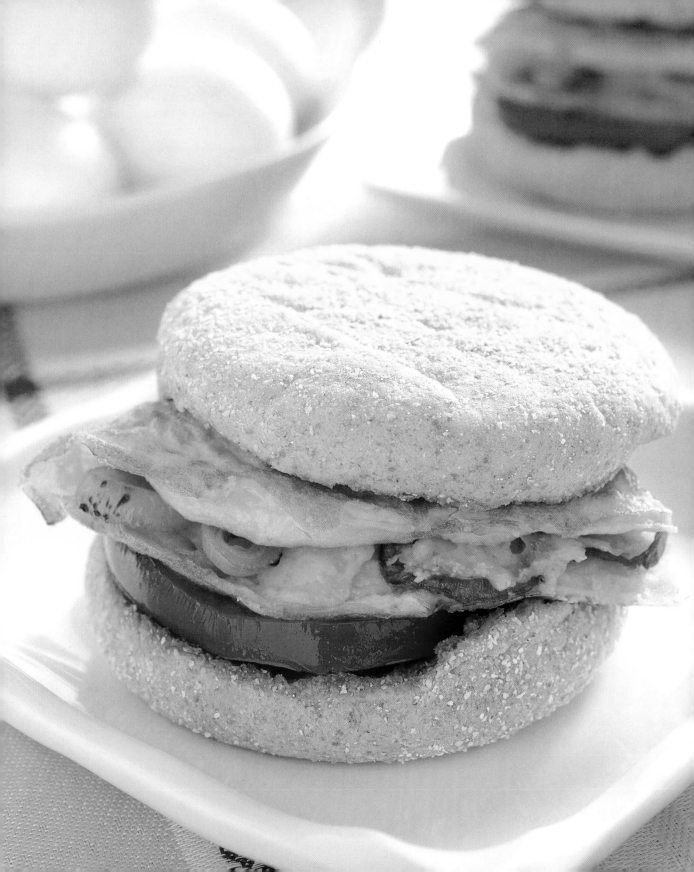

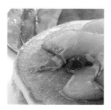

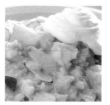

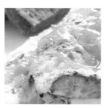

breakfast

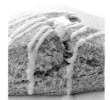

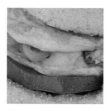

◀ *Egg Muffin Sandwiches, page 22*

SMOOTHIES AND CEREALS

PANCAKES AND WAFFLES

MUFFINS, SCONES, AND MORE

EGG AND MEAT DISHES

Watermelon-Strawberry Smoothies

Prep Time: 10 minutes

For a slushy summery treat, freeze the watermelon and strawberry chunks before you blend them.

   4   cups watermelon chunks
   1   quart strawberries, hulled
   2   teaspoons honey
   2   cups low-fat vanilla yogurt
   4   teaspoons blanched chopped almonds

In blender combine watermelon, strawberries, honey, yogurt, and almonds. Process until smooth. Divide among 4 glasses.

Makes 4 servings

to complete the meal   Per serving: 1 slice whole grain toast with 1 tablespoon peanut butter

COMPLETE MEAL SERVING
372 calories / 12 g total fat / 107 calories from fat / 29% calories from fat
6 mg cholesterol / 246 mg sodium / 10 g carbohydrate / 10 g fiber / 41 g sugars / 14 g protein

moving forward
Changing your lifestyle isn't easy. Be prepared for good days and bad days and don't give up.

Mixed Berry-Yogurt Smoothies

Prep Time: 10 minutes

Whether you like your drinks thick like a frozen drink, or creamier, like a smoothie, you can get either result. For a thinner smoothie drink, allow the frozen berries to stand at room temperature for about 10 minutes. For the thicker version, use the berries straight from the freezer.

1	cup frozen blueberries
1	cup frozen raspberries
1	cup frozen strawberries
1	cup low-fat vanilla yogurt
¼	cup reduced-fat sour cream
2	tablespoons frozen orange juice concentrate
1	teaspoon crystallized ginger

In blender combine blueberries, raspberries, strawberries, yogurt, sour cream, orange juice concentrate, and ginger. Process until smooth. Divide between 2 glasses.

Makes 2 servings

to complete the meal Per serving: 1 slice seven-grain toast with 1 teaspoon
trans-fat-free canola margarine

COMPLETE MEAL SERVING
372 calories / 11 g total fat / 97 calories from fat / 25% calories from fat
18 mg cholesterol / 255 mg sodium / 62 g carbohydrate / 10 g fiber / 41 g sugars / 11 g protein

Apple-Cinnamon Oatmeal

Prep Time: 5 minutes ■ Cook Time: 8 minutes

Cooked in juice with fruit and spices, this oatmeal is like eating a steaming bowl of apple crisp for breakfast.

1	cup apple juice
½	cup cranberry juice cocktail
⅛	teaspoon salt
1	cup rolled oats
1	large apple, cored and chopped (about 1¼ cups)
¼	cup low-fat (1%) milk
2	tablespoons packed brown sugar
¾	teaspoon apple pie spice or ground cinnamon
½	cup chopped pecans, toasted

1 In medium saucepan bring apple juice, cranberry cocktail, and salt to boiling. Stir in oats and apple; cook over medium heat for 5 minutes, stirring occasionally. Stir in milk, brown sugar, and apple pie spice; cook for 1 minute.

2 Spoon into 4 bowls and sprinkle with pecans.

Makes 4 servings

to complete the meal   Per serving: ¼ cup low-fat (1%) milk

COMPLETE MEAL SERVING
376 calories / 13 g total fat / 115 calories from fat / 29% calories from fat
5 mg cholesterol / 214 mg sodium / 55 g carbohydrate / 5 g fiber / 38 g sugars / 14 g protein

Peach-Almond Oatmeal

Prep Time: 3 minutes ■ Cook Time: 8 minutes

Research has found that people who eat oatmeal as part of their diet and exercise programs lose more pounds and inches than those who don't. Here's a tasty variation to try.

- 4   cups water
- 2   teaspoons almond extract
- 2   cups rolled oats
- ¼   teaspoon salt
- 2   cups chopped fresh peaches or canned peaches in juice, drained and diced
- ¾   cup sliced natural almonds
- ¼   cup low-fat vanilla yogurt

1 In medium saucepan bring the water and almond extract to boiling; add oats and salt. Reduce heat, cover, and simmer for 5 minutes, stirring occasionally, until water is almost all absorbed. Fold in peaches and almonds.

2 Divide among 4 bowls. Top each with 1 tablespoon of the yogurt.

Makes 4 servings

COMPLETE MEAL SERVING
341 calories / 12 g total fat / 106 calories from fat / 30% calories from fat
1 mg cholesterol / 167 mg sodium / 48 g carbohydrate / 7 g fiber / 18 g sugars / 11 g protein

moving forward
Don't skip meals. This could lead to binge eating and treatment effects.

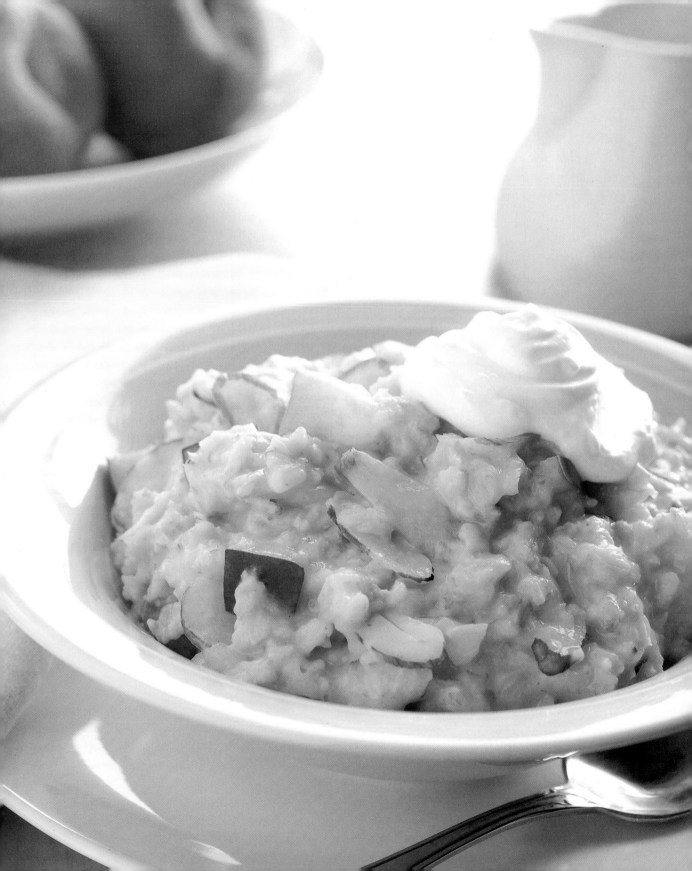

Fruit and Nut Granola

Prep Time: 10 minutes ■ Cook Time: 48 minutes

Here's granola made the old-fashioned way with pure maple syrup and lots of nuts, fruit, and other delectable ingredients. For the best results, use old-fashioned (not quick) oats, which will bake into crisp, golden granola.

	Nonstick cooking spray
4	cups rolled oats
½	cup slivered almonds
½	cup chopped pecans
½	cup packed brown sugar
¼	cup maple syrup or honey
¼	cup water
¼	teaspoon salt
2	teaspoons vanilla
⅓	cup chopped dried apples
⅓	cup dried cranberries

1 Preheat oven to 300°F. Lightly spray jelly-roll pan with nonstick cooking spray.

2 In large bowl combine oats, almonds, and pecans.

3 In small saucepan bring brown sugar, maple syrup, water, and salt to boiling. Remove from heat and stir in vanilla. Stir sugar mixture into oat mixture and toss until evenly coated. Evenly spread on prepared pan.

4 Bake for 45 minutes, stirring every 15 minutes. Remove pan from oven and stir in apples and cranberries. Place on rack to cool completely.

5 Store granola in airtight container at room temperature.

Makes nine ⅔-cup servings

to complete the meal Per serving: ⅓ cup reduced-fat (2%) milk

COMPLETE MEAL SERVING
376 calories / 12 g total fat / 107 calories from fat / 28% calories from fat
9 mg cholesterol / 155 mg sodium / 57 g carbohydrate / 5 g fiber / 29 g sugars / 12 g protein

Crunchy Berry Breakfast

Prep Time: 5 minutes ■ Cook Time: 4 minutes

Chewy, chunky, nutty, and fruity describes this breakfast that's sure to make a frequent appearance on your breakfast table.

1	cup plain low-fat yogurt
½	cup prepared vanilla pudding
¾	cup rolled oats
1	tablespoon honey
1	cup mixed berries (blueberries, raspberries, blackberries, and cranberries)
½	cup chopped walnuts

1 In small bowl mix yogurt and pudding. Set aside.

2 In medium skillet over medium heat toast oats, stirring frequently, for 1 minute or until lightly browned. Drizzle with honey; cook for 3 minutes or until oats are crispy and lightly toasted.

3 Divide ½ cup of the oats among 4 parfait glasses or small bowls. Reserve remaining oats. Divide half of the berries over oats. Sprinkle each with 2 tablespoons of the walnuts. Divide yogurt mixture over berries. Top with remaining berries and remaining oats.

Makes 4 servings

to complete the meal Per serving: 1 slice whole grain toast with 1 tablespoon strawberry all-fruit spread

COMPLETE MEAL SERVING
339 calories / 10 g total fat / 89 calories from fat / 26% calories from fat
6 mg cholesterol / 230 mg sodium / 53 g carbohydrate / 5 g fiber / 26 g sugars / 11 g protein

moving forward
Don't consider exercise lost time. Taking care of yourself should be a priority.

Whole Grain Waffles with Berry Syrup

Prep Time: 10 minutes ■ Cook Time: 20 minutes

Adding cream of tartar to the batter creates waffles that are light and fluffy on the inside and deliciously crisp on the outside. Then they're smothered with a fresh-tasting berry syrup that's loaded with good-for-you antioxidants.

Waffles

- 1 cup all-purpose flour
- 1 cup whole wheat pastry flour
- 1 tablespoon sugar
- 1 teaspoon cream of tartar
- ½ teaspoon baking soda
- ½ teaspoon salt
- 2 eggs
- 1¾ cups reduced-fat (2%) milk
- 2 tablespoons vegetable oil

Syrup

- 1 12-ounce package frozen assorted berries, such as strawberries, raspberries, blackberries, and blueberries
- ½ cup maple syrup
- ⅓ cup orange juice
- 6 tablespoons chopped walnuts

1 For waffles, preheat oven to 200°F and preheat waffle iron.

2 In large bowl combine all-purpose flour, pastry flour, sugar, cream of tartar, baking soda, and salt until blended.

3 In medium bowl whisk together eggs, milk, and oil. Stir milk mixture into flour mixture just until blended. Cook waffles in batches until done. Place waffles on ovensafe plate; keep warm in oven.

4 Meanwhile, for berry syrup, in small saucepan combine berries, maple syrup, and orange juice. Bring to boiling. Reduce heat to medium; simmer for 3 minutes. Remove from heat; keep warm.

5 Place 2 waffles on each of 6 large plates. Divide berry syrup over waffles. Sprinkle each set of waffles with 1 tablespoon of the walnuts.

Makes 6 servings

COMPLETE MEAL SERVING
404 calories / 13 g total fat / 117 calories from fat / 29% calories from fat
76 mg cholesterol / 354 mg sodium / 63 g carbohydrate / 5 g fiber / 26 g sugars / 10 g protein

Ricotta Pancakes with Dried Fruit Sauce

Prep Time: 10 minutes ■ Cook Time: 20 minutes

Dried fruit adds a healthy punch of concentrated flavor and sweetness to the sauce, while the protein-packed ricotta cheese in this simple-to-make batter yields perfect pancakes that are moist, yet light. The contrast is scrumptious.

Sauce		
1	cup chopped assorted dried fruit, such as plums, apples, apricots, peaches, and pears
1	cup apple cider
¼	cup packed brown sugar
¼	teaspoon ground ginger

Pancakes		
1	cup all-purpose flour
¼	cup granulated sugar
1	teaspoon baking powder
½	teaspoon baking soda
½	teaspoon salt
2	eggs
1	cup part-skim ricotta cheese
½	cup low-fat (1%) milk
1	teaspoon vanilla
	Nonstick cooking spray
½	cup chopped pecans

1 For sauce, in small saucepan combine dried fruit, cider, brown sugar, and ginger. Bring to boiling. Reduce heat to medium; simmer for 3 minutes. Remove from heat; keep warm.

2 Meanwhile, for pancakes, in large bowl combine flour, granulated sugar, baking powder, baking soda, and salt until blended.

3 In medium bowl whisk together eggs, ricotta cheese, milk, and vanilla. Stir ricotta mixture into flour mixture just until blended.

4 Preheat oven to 200°F. Lightly spray large nonstick skillet with nonstick cooking spray and place over medium heat until hot. For each pancake, pour about ¼ cup of the batter into skillet. Cook for 3 minutes or until bubbles appear on top and edges are barely dry. Turn pancakes and cook for 1 minute or until centers spring back when touched. Place pancakes on ovensafe plate and keep warm in oven. Repeat with remaining batter, lightly coating skillet with nonstick cooking spray as needed.

5 Place 2 pancakes on each of 6 large plates. Divide fruit sauce over pancakes. Top each set of pancakes with 1 heaping tablespoon of the pecans.

Makes 6 servings

COMPLETE MEAL SERVING
380 calories / 12 g total fat / 111 calories from fat / 29% calories from fat
85 mg cholesterol / 575 mg sodium / 58 g carbohydrate / 3 g fiber / 36 g sugars / 11 g protein

Buttermilk Pancakes with Sauteed Pears

Prep Time: 10 minutes ■ Cook Time: 15 minutes

Easy and elegant, sauteed pears transform basic-but-delicious buttermilk pancakes into a dish with lots of "Wow!" factor plus a healthy dose of vitamin C and fiber. You'll never miss the syrup.

Pears
- 1½ tablespoons trans-fat-free canola margarine
- 3 pears, peeled, cored, and sliced
- 2 tablespoons sugar
- 1 teaspoon vanilla

Pancakes
- ¾ cup all-purpose flour
- ¾ cup whole wheat pastry flour
- 2 tablespoons ground flaxseeds
- 1 tablespoon sugar
- 1 teaspoon baking powder
- ½ teaspoon baking soda
- ¼ teaspoon salt
- 2 eggs or ½ cup egg substitute
- 1½ cups reduced-fat buttermilk
- Nonstick cooking spray

1 For pears, in large nonstick skillet melt margarine over medium-high heat and cook pears with sugar and vanilla, stirring occasionally, for 10 minutes or until caramelized and tender. Remove skillet from heat and keep warm.

2 Meanwhile, for pancakes, in large bowl combine all-purpose flour, pastry flour, flaxseeds, sugar, baking powder, baking soda, and salt until blended.

3 In medium bowl whisk together eggs and buttermilk. Stir milk mixture into flour mixture just until blended.

4 Preheat oven to 200°F. Lightly spray large nonstick skillet with nonstick cooking spray and place over medium heat until hot. For each pancake, pour about ¼ cup of the batter into skillet. Cook for 3 minutes or until bubbles appear on top and edges are barely dry. Turn pancakes and cook for 1 minute or until centers spring back when touched. Place pancakes on ovensafe plate and keep warm in oven. Repeat with remaining batter, lightly coating skillet with nonstick cooking spray as needed.

5 Place 2 pancakes on each of 6 large plates. Divide pears over pancakes.

Makes 6 servings

to complete the meal   Per serving: 2 ounces broiled Canadian bacon

COMPLETE MEAL SERVING
359 calories / 11 g total fat / 97 calories from fat / 27% calories from fat
100 mg cholesterol / 1,095 mg sodium / 46 g carbohydrate / 5 g fiber / 19 g sugars / 19 g protein

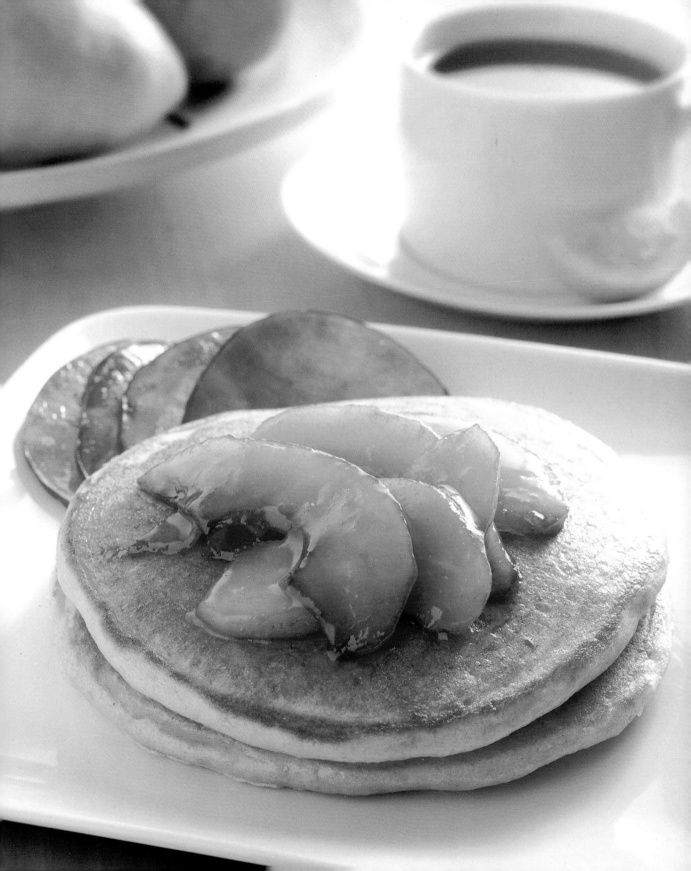

Strawberry-Stuffed French Toast

Prep Time: 15 minutes ■ Cook Time: 14 minutes

A thick, hearty slice of whole wheat bread with warm fruit filling is a great way to start the day. For perfect slices, place a whole loaf on its side and lightly "saw" through the bread with a sharp serrated knife.

2	ounces ⅓-less-fat cream cheese (Neufchâtel), softened
¼	cup strawberry preserves
4	4x3x1-inch slices whole wheat bread
2	eggs
1	egg white
½	cup low-fat (1%) milk
2	tablespoons granulated sugar
1	teaspoon vanilla
	Nonstick cooking spray
2	teaspoons trans-fat-free canola margarine
2	cups fresh sliced strawberries
4	teaspoons powdered sugar

1 In small bowl combine cream cheese and preserves until blended. Cut a slit in each slice of bread from one side, being careful not to cut through the other 3 sides, to form a pocket. Evenly stuff 1 heaping tablespoon of the cream cheese mixture into each pocket.

2 In 11x7-inch baking dish, whisk together eggs, egg white, milk, granulated sugar, and vanilla. Arrange stuffed bread slices in dish; let stand for 10 minutes, or until egg mixture is absorbed, turning once.

3 Lightly spray large nonstick skillet with nonstick cooking spray and place over medium heat until hot. Add 1 teaspoon of the margarine and cook 2 slices of the French toast for 7 minutes or until brown, turning once. Repeat with remaining 1 teaspoon margarine and 2 slices of the French toast.

4 Place 1 slice of French toast on each of 4 plates. Top each with ½ cup of the strawberries and 1 teaspoon of the powdered sugar.

Makes 4 servings

COMPLETE MEAL SERVING
291 calories / 10 g total fat / 29 calories from fat / 29% calories from fat
120 mg cholesterol / 282 mg sodium / 43 g carbohydrate / 4 g fiber / 28 g sugars / 10 g protein

Raspberry–Sour Cream Muffins

Prep Time: 10 minutes ■ Bake Time: 18 minutes

Whole wheat pastry flour and sour cream give these muffins a tender, cakelike texture. To get that fresh-from-the-oven flavor the next day, sprinkle a muffin with a few drops of water, loosely wrap in foil, and heat in a 350°F oven for 8 minutes or until moist and warm.

Nonstick cooking spray
1 cup all-purpose flour
1 cup whole wheat pastry flour
1 cup sugar
2 teaspoons baking powder
1 teaspoon baking soda
½ teaspoon salt
2 eggs
1 cup reduced-fat sour cream
¼ cup low-fat (1%) milk
¼ cup light olive oil
1½ teaspoons vanilla
2 cups fresh raspberries
½ cup dried blueberries

1 Preheat oven to 400°F. Lightly spray 12-cup muffin pan with nonstick cooking spray.

2 In large bowl combine all-purpose flour, pastry flour, sugar, baking powder, baking soda, and salt until blended.

3 In medium bowl whisk together eggs, sour cream, milk, oil, and vanilla. Stir egg mixture into flour mixture just until blended. Gently stir in raspberries and blueberries.

4 Divide batter among muffin cups. Bake for 18 minutes or until wooden toothpick inserted in centers comes out clean. Cool in pan on wire rack for 10 minutes. Remove muffins to rack and cool completely.

Makes 12 servings

to complete the meal   Per serving: 1 teaspoon trans-fat-free canola margarine ■ 1 cup fat-free (skim) milk

COMPLETE MEAL SERVING
374 calories / 12 g total fat / 111 calories from fat / 30% calories from fat
48 mg cholesterol / 446 mg sodium / 53 g carbohydrate / 3 g fiber / 32 g sugars / 13 g protein

Apple-Spice Muffins

Prep Time: 10 minutes ■ Bake Time: 18 minutes

If you don't have apple pie spice on hand, make your own by mixing together 2 teaspoons ground cinnamon, ½ teaspoon nutmeg, and ¼ teaspoon each allspice and ground cardamom.

	Nonstick cooking spray
1	cup all-purpose flour
1	cup whole wheat pastry flour
¾	cup packed brown sugar
2	teaspoons baking powder
1	teaspoon baking soda
1	tablespoon apple pie spice
½	teaspoon salt
2	eggs
1	cup low-fat buttermilk
¼	cup light olive oil
2	cups peeled, shredded apple (2)
½	cup chopped pecans
3	tablespoons cinnamon sugar

1 Preheat oven to 400°F. Lightly spray 12-cup muffin pan with nonstick cooking spray.

2 In large bowl combine all-purpose flour, pastry flour, brown sugar, baking powder, baking soda, apple pie spice, and salt until blended.

3 In medium bowl whisk together eggs, buttermilk, and oil. Stir egg mixture into flour mixture just until blended. Gently stir in apple and pecans.

4 Divide batter among muffin cups. Evenly sprinkle tops of muffins with cinnamon sugar.

5 Bake for 18 minutes or until wooden toothpick inserted in centers comes out clean. Cool in pan on wire rack for 10 minutes. Remove muffins to rack and cool completely.

Makes 12 servings

to complete the meal   Per serving: 4 teaspoons fat-free cream cheese ■ 1 cup fat-free (skim) milk

COMPLETE MEAL SERVING
350 calories / 10 g total fat / 91 calories from fat / 26% calories from fat
43 mg cholesterol / 537 mg sodium / 50 g carbohydrate / 3 g fiber / 32 g sugars / 15 g protein

Banana-Bran Muffins

Prep Time: 10 minutes ▪ Bake Time: 20 minutes

There's no need to toss out overripe bananas. Use them in an uncommonly good bran muffin that comes together in a snap. Want to save some for later? Double-wrap the muffins in plastic and freeze them for up to 1 month.

Nonstick cooking spray
1   cup wheat bran
1   cup reduced-fat (2%) milk
1   large egg, beaten
3   tablespoons olive oil
1   cup all-purpose flour
2   teaspoons baking powder
½   teaspoon salt
1   cup mashed ripe banana (2)
½   cup honey
¾   cup chopped walnuts

1 Preheat oven to 375°F. Lightly spray 12-cup muffin pan with nonstick cooking spray.

2 In medium bowl combine bran, milk, egg, and oil; let stand 5 minutes.

3 In large bowl combine flour, baking powder, and salt until blended. Stir banana and honey into milk mixture; stir milk mixture into flour mixture just until blended. Stir in walnuts.

4 Divide batter among muffin cups. Bake for 20 minutes or until wooden toothpick inserted in centers comes out clean. Cool in pan on wire rack for 10 minutes. Remove muffins to rack and cool completely.

Makes 12 servings

to complete the meal   Per serving: ½ large pink grapefruit ▪ 1 cup fat-free (skim) milk

COMPLETE MEAL SERVING
341 calories / 10 g total fat / 93 calories from fat / 26% calories from fat
25 mg cholesterol / 304 mg sodium / 53 g carbohydrate / 4 g fiber / 40 g sugars / 14 g protein

Orange Scones

Prep Time: 15 minutes ■ Bake Time: 15 minutes

Fragrant and lightly sweet, scones are perfect for breakfast with a cup of tea. The trick to good soft scones: The less you handle the dough, the better. Not all scones are created equally. This recipe allows you to enjoy these tasty bites but avoid purchased scones as they are loaded with fat and calories.

	Nonstick cooking spray
½	cup low-fat (1%) milk
1	egg
1	tablespoon grated orange zest
1	teaspoon vanilla
1½	cups all-purpose flour
½	cup whole wheat pastry flour
¼	cup ground pecans
¼	cup granulated sugar
2	teaspoons baking powder
½	teaspoon salt
¼	cup chilled trans-fat-free canola margarine, cut into small pieces
¼	cup powdered sugar
2	teaspoons fresh orange juice

1 Preheat oven to 425°F. Lightly spray baking sheet with nonstick cooking spray. In medium bowl whisk together milk, egg, zest, and vanilla.

2 In large bowl combine all-purpose flour, pastry flour, pecans, granulated sugar, baking powder, and salt until blended. Using pastry blender or two knives, cut in margarine until size of coarse meal. Add milk mixture to flour mixture and stir until dough just holds together. Using floured hands, knead dough gently against sides of bowl 10 times or until smooth ball of dough forms.

3 On floured surface, pat dough into 7-inch circle. Cut dough into 10 wedges. Separate wedges and arrange on prepared baking sheet. Bake for 15 minutes or until golden. Remove to rack to cool.

4 In small bowl whisk together powdered sugar and orange juice until smooth. Drizzle over scones.

Makes 10 servings

to complete the meal   Per serving: 1 cup low-fat (1%) milk

COMPLETE MEAL SERVING
291 calories / 10 g total fat / 86 calories from fat / 30% calories from fat
10 mg cholesterol / 361 mg sodium / 40 g carbohydrate / 2 g fiber / 20 g sugars / 11 g protein

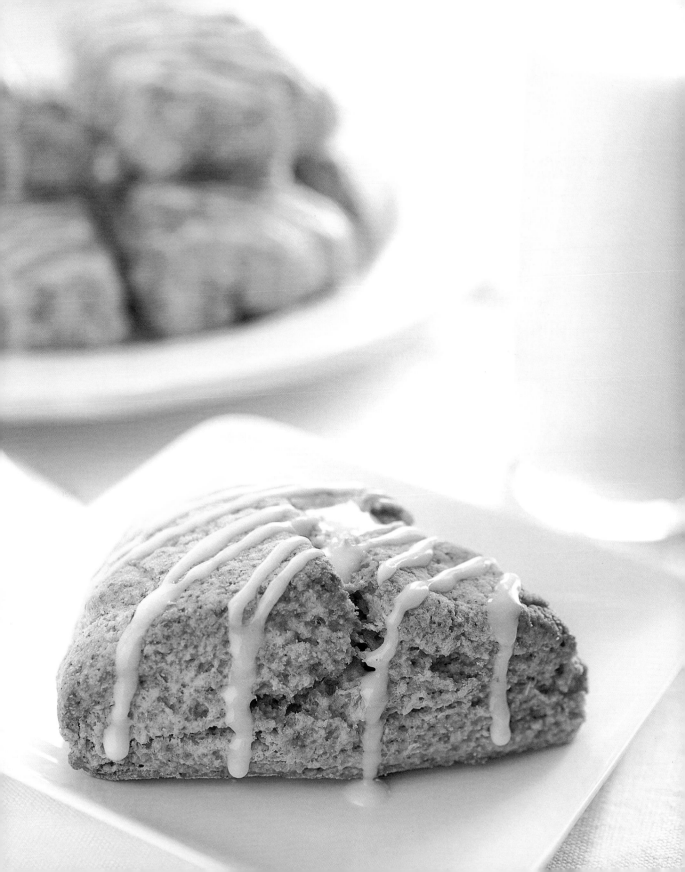

Fruit-Topped Breakfast Pizza

Prep Time: 10 minutes ■ Bake Time: 12 minutes

A pizza topped with a feast of vitamin-rich fresh fruit creates a smashingly colorful centerpiece for your breakfast table that tastes as luscious as it looks. Family and friends will dive right in.

Nonstick cooking spray

1 13.8-ounce tube refrigerated pizza crust

1 large egg, beaten

2 teaspoons cinnamon sugar

1 cup part-skim ricotta cheese

¼ cup low-fat vanilla yogurt

3 cups cut-up fresh fruit such as strawberries, raspberries, blueberries, kiwifruit, and cantaloupe

⅓ cup sweetened flaked coconut, toasted

1 Preheat oven to 400°F. Lightly spray baking sheet with nonstick cooking spray.

2 Unroll crust onto prepared baking sheet and press into 14×9-inch rectangle. Brush crust with egg; sprinkle with cinnamon sugar. Bake for 12 minutes or until golden brown. Remove from oven and let cool.

3 In small bowl combine ricotta cheese and yogurt. Spread cheese mixture over cooled crust, leaving a ½-inch border around sides. Evenly top cheese mixture with fruit; sprinkle with coconut.

Makes 8 servings

to complete the meal   Per serving: ¾ cup reduced-fat (2%) milk

COMPLETE MEAL SERVING
321 calories / 10 g total fat / 87 calories from fat / 27% calories from fat
51 mg cholesterol / 478 mg sodium / 43 g carbohydrate / 3 g fiber / 19 g sugars / 16 g protein

Scrambled Egg Cups

Prep Time: 15 minutes ■ Cook Time: 12 minutes

Tender, crisp phyllo cups filled with mushroom scrambled eggs make a great breakfast treat. They're delicious for the family yet lovely enough to serve to guests. Prepare the phyllo cups ahead and store them in an airtight container for up to 2 days.

	Nonstick cooking spray
8	sheets phyllo dough, thawed according to package directions
½	cup chopped fresh herbs such as parsley, oregano, basil, and/or thyme
2	eggs
4	egg whites
3	cups sliced shiitake mushrooms
2	tablespoons trans-fat-free canola margarine
½	cup sliced green onion (4)

1 Preheat oven to 350°F. Lightly spray 8 cups of a 12-cup muffin pan with nonstick cooking spray.

2 For each phyllo cup, lay 1 phyllo sheet on work surface and cut into quarters. Spray all quarters lightly with nonstick cooking spray. Sprinkle 3 of the quarters lightly with 1 teaspoon of the herbs each. Stack quarters, ending with plain quarter (the one with no herbs) on top. Press stack into muffin cup. Repeat with remaining 7 phyllo sheets and herbs.

3 Bake phyllo cups for 12 minutes or until lightly golden. Place on rack to cool.

4 Meanwhile, in small bowl whisk together eggs and egg whites. In large nonstick skillet over medium-high heat cook mushrooms in hot margarine, stirring occasionally, for 5 minutes or until tender. Add green onion and cook 1 minute. Add egg mixture and cook, stirring occasionally, for 3 minutes or until eggs are set. Divide egg mixture into phyllo cups.

Makes 4 servings

to complete the meal   Per serving: 1 small banana

COMPLETE MEAL SERVING
330 calories / 11 g total fat / 99 calories from fat / 29% calories from fat
106 mg cholesterol / 327 mg sodium / 48 g carbohydrate / 4 g fiber / 21 g sugars / 12 g protein

Egg Muffin Sandwiches

Prep Time: 5 minutes ■ Cook Time: 10 minutes

The calories, saturated fat, and sodium of a traditional egg sandwich are slashed here by adding veggies and Parmesan cheese for flavor and leaving out the standard slice of high-fat, high-sodium meat.

 2 whole wheat English muffins, split and toasted
 2 eggs
 4 egg whites
 ⅛ teaspoon ground black pepper
    Nonstick cooking spray
 ½ cup thinly sliced shallot (2)
 2 ½-inch-thick slices tomato
 ¼ cup grated Parmesan cheese

1 Place 1 English muffin half on each of 2 plates; set aside.

2 In small bowl whisk together eggs, egg whites, and pepper.

3 In large nonstick skillet lightly coated with nonstick cooking spray cook shallot over medium-high heat, stirring occasionally, for 3 minutes or until lightly brown. Remove shallots from skillet and set aside. Add tomato slices to skillet; cook for 2 minutes, turning once. Place tomato slices on muffins.

4 Add eggs to skillet, tilting pan to cover. Cook for 3 minutes or until eggs begin to set. Sprinkle with cheese and shallots. Fold omelet in half; cover and cook for 2 minutes or until eggs are set. Cut omelet into 2 equal pieces. Place 1 half on each tomato slice. Top with remaining English muffin halves.

Makes 2 servings

COMPLETE MEAL SERVING
323 calories / 10 g total fat / 86 calories from fat / 26% calories from fat
220 mg cholesterol / 788 mg sodium / 37 g carbohydrate / 5 g fiber / 6 g sugars / 25 g protein

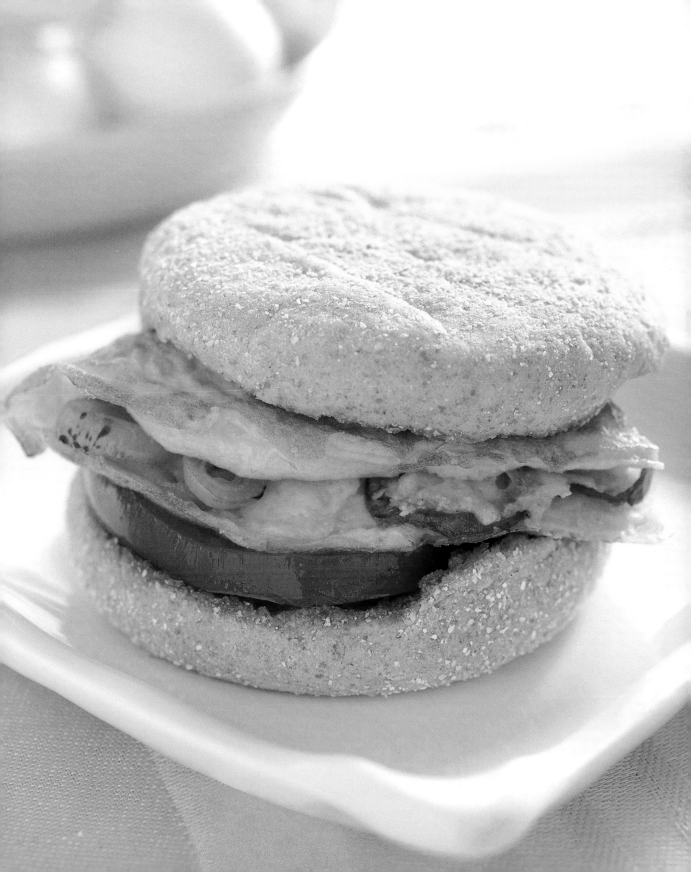

Chilaquiles en Salsa Verde

Prep Time: 10 minutes ■ Cook Time: 11 minutes

Unlike nachos, which are served as a crispy snack, chilaquiles are a main dish—traditionally eaten at breakfast—and are not served until the tortilla chips are thoroughly soaked and softened by the salsa.

	Nonstick cooking spray
8	6-inch corn tortillas
2	8-ounce cans mild salsa verde
½	cup reduced-fat sour cream
½	avocado, peeled, pitted, and mashed
¼	cup shredded low-fat white cheddar cheese
4	to 5 sprigs fresh cilantro

1 Preheat oven to 350°F. Lightly spray baking sheet with nonstick cooking spray.

2 Lightly spray tortillas with cooking spray. Cut each tortilla into 6 wedges. Place tortilla pieces on baking sheet and bake for 5 minutes or until golden brown.

3 In large saucepan heat salsa on medium heat for 3 minutes or until hot. Fold in baked tortilla pieces and sour cream. Cook for 5 minutes or until tortillas are soft. Top with avocado, cheese, and cilantro.

Makes 4 servings

to complete the meal   Per serving: Cantaloupe wedge (⅛ of large melon)

COMPLETE MEAL SERVING
285 calories / 10 g total fat / 88 calories from fat / 30% calories from fat
17 mg cholesterol / 534 mg sodium / 44 g carbohydrate / 5 g fiber / 12 g sugars / 7 g protein

Lite Machaca Omelet

Prep Time: 5 minutes ■ Cook Time: 5 minutes

Mexican machaca dishes are traditionally prepared with spicy dried beef. In this leaner version, lean chicken breast cuts the fat but keeps the kick. Make it hot or not!

5	egg whites
1	egg
1	cup shredded cooked chicken breast
3	cups baby spinach
¼	cup sliced mushrooms
2	tablespoons hot sauce
1½	teaspoons olive oil

1 In large bowl whisk together egg whites, egg, chicken, spinach, mushrooms, and hot sauce.

2 In large nonstick skillet cook egg mixture in hot oil over medium heat, tilting skillet to cover. Cook for 3 minutes or until eggs start to set; flip omelet; cook for 2 minutes or until set.

Makes 4 servings

to complete the meal   Per serving: 1 slice whole wheat toast with 1 teaspoon trans-fat-free canola margarine ■ 1 large orange

COMPLETE MEAL SERVING
316 calories / 10 g total fat / 90 calories from fat / 27% calories from fat
83 mg cholesterol / 482 mg sodium / 37 g carbohydrate / 7 g fiber / 19 g sugars / 22 g protein

moving forward
Don't get discouraged if things seem to be taking a while. You're on your way.

Broccoli-Cheese Omelet

Prep Time: 5 minutes ■ Cook Time: 11 minutes

Here's a great way to use leftover steamed broccoli from yesterday's dinner for a protein-packed breakfast that's ready in minutes. Instead of the frozen broccoli, chop the leftover broccoli to measure 1¼ cups.

	Nonstick cooking spray
1	cup chopped onion
1	10-ounce box frozen chopped broccoli, thawed, squeezed, and drained
6	egg whites
1	egg
¼	cup low-fat (1%) milk
⅓	cup shredded reduced-fat cheddar cheese

1 In large nonstick skillet lightly coated with nonstick cooking spray cook onion over medium-high heat, stirring occasionally, for 3 minutes or until tender and lightly brown. Add broccoli and cook for 1 minute. Reduce heat to medium.

2 In medium bowl whisk together egg whites, egg, and milk. Pour egg mixture over vegetables. Cook, lifting eggs at edges and tilting to cook egg mixture on top, for 5 minutes or until bottom starts to brown and eggs are almost set. Fold omelet in half; cook 2 minutes or until eggs are set. Remove skillet from heat, sprinkle with cheese, cover, and set aside for 1 minute to melt cheese.

Makes 2 servings

to complete the meal   Per serving: 1 slice whole wheat toast with 1 teaspoon trans-fat-free canola margarine

COMPLETE MEAL SERVING
306 calories / 10 g total fat / 93 calories from fat / 29% calories from fat
121 mg cholesterol / 563 mg sodium / 30 g carbohydrate / 8 g fiber / 11 g sugars / 27 g protein

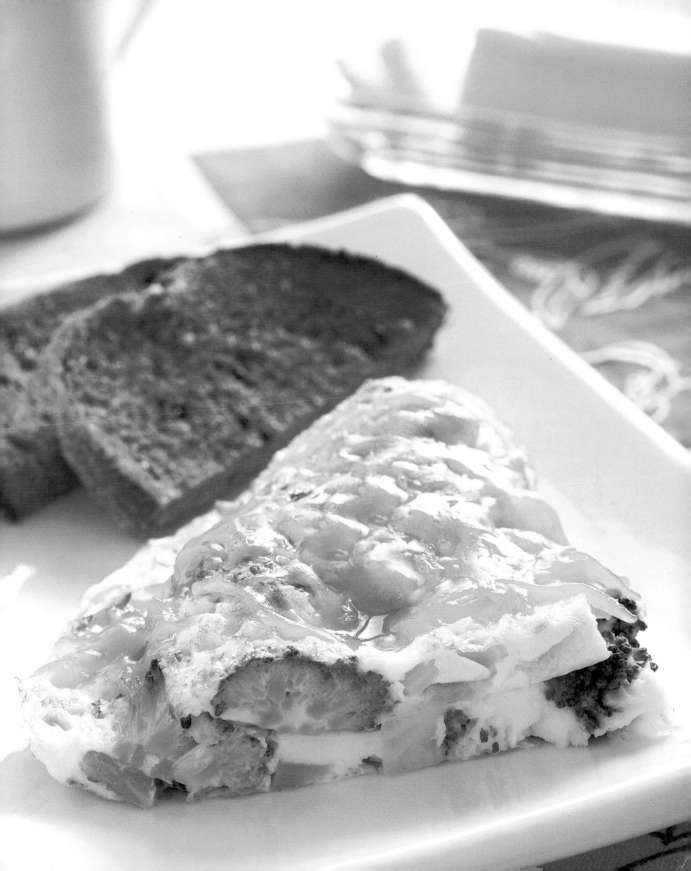

Cheese Grits with Ham

Prep Time: 5 minutes ■ Cook Time: 10 minutes

There's a reason why Southerners love grits. Made from coarsely ground corn, it's a simple, wholesome, easily digested food that pairs equally well with both savory and sweet flavors. This recipe includes a little of both.

1½ cups low-fat (1%) milk
1½ cups water
¾ cup uncooked quick-cooking grits
¼ teaspoon salt
1 cup shredded 75% reduced-fat cheddar cheese (4 ounces)
4 ounces thinly sliced ham, cut into 1-inch-long thin strips
2 tablespoons maple syrup

1 In medium saucepan bring milk and water to boiling over medium-high heat. Slowly stir in grits and salt. Reduce heat to low; cover and cook, stirring occasionally, for 7 minutes or until thickened.

2 Remove from heat and stir in cheese until melted. Divide among 4 bowls. Divide ham over each and drizzle each with ½ tablespoon of the maple syrup.

Makes 4 servings

to complete the meal Per serving: 1 slice whole wheat toast with 1 teaspoon trans-fat-free canola margarine

COMPLETE MEAL SERVING
393 calories / 13 g total fat / 117 calories from fat / 29% calories from fat
31 mg cholesterol / 933 mg sodium / 51 g carbohydrate / 2 g fiber / 12 g sugars / 20 g protein

moving forward
Schedule exercise into your day like an appointment you can't miss.

Soul Frittata

Prep Time: 5 minutes ■ Cook Time: 19 minutes

Kale, a member of the cabbage family, is a traditional ingredient in Southern cooking. An excellent source of vitamins A, C, and K, kale will add great flavor and good nutrition to your meals.

8	egg whites
2	eggs
½	teaspoon salt
¼	teaspoon ground black pepper
5	strips turkey bacon, chopped
1	tablespoon olive oil
¼	cup chopped onion
¼	cup chopped red sweet pepper
¼	cup chopped yellow sweet pepper
4	cups chopped kale
2	tablespoons water
½	cup shredded low-fat cheddar cheese

1 Preheat broiler.

2 In large bowl whisk together egg whites, eggs, salt, and black pepper.

3 In large broilerproof skillet cook bacon in hot oil over medium heat for 3 minutes or until brown. Remove to bowl with eggs. Add onion and sweet peppers; cook for 2 minutes. With slotted spoon remove to bowl with eggs.

4 Add half of the kale to skillet and toss until starting to wilt. Add remaining kale; cook and stir for 2 minutes. Add the water, cover, and cook for 5 minutes or until tender and dry.

5 Pour egg mixture over kale in skillet. Cook over medium heat for 5 minutes. As mixture sets, run a spatula around skillet edge, lifting egg mixture so uncooked portion flows underneath. Continue cooking and lifting edges until egg mixture is almost set. (The surface will be moist.) Reduce heat as necessary to prevent overcooking.

6 Broil 4 to 5 inches from heat for 2 minutes or until top is set. Sprinkle cheese over frittata.

Makes 4 servings

to complete the meal   Per serving: 1 slice whole wheat toast with 1 teaspoon apple all-fruit spread

COMPLETE MEAL SERVING
287 calories / 10 g total fat / 87 calories from fat / 30% calories from fat
114 mg cholesterol / 619 mg sodium / 29 g carbohydrate / 4 g fiber / 6 g sugars / 21 g protein

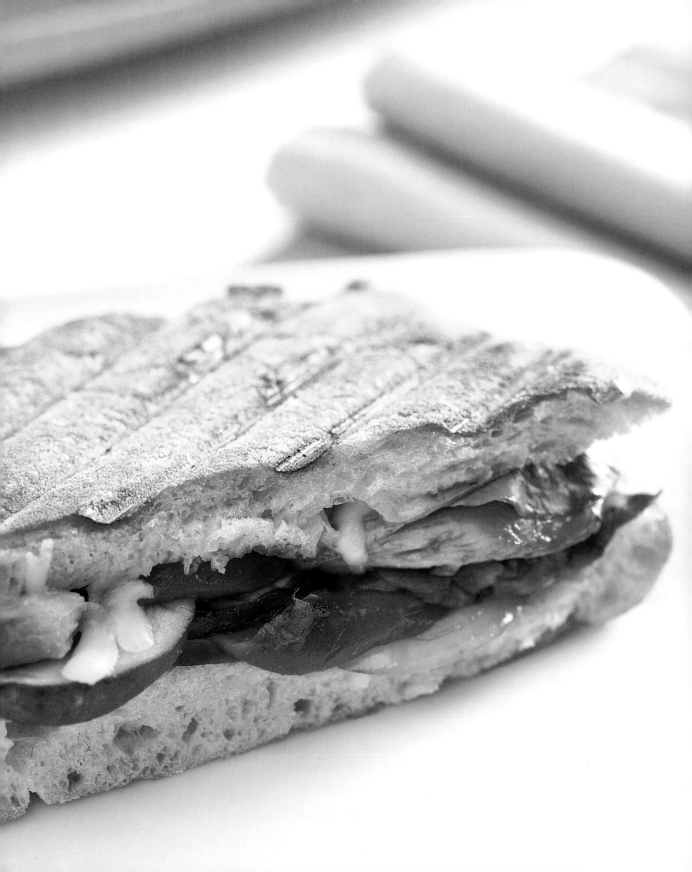

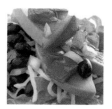

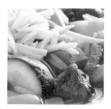

lunch

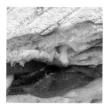

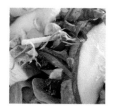

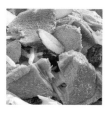

◄ *Roasted Red Pepper and*
Chicken Panini, page 68

Chicken Tortilla Soup

Prep Time: 9 minutes ■ Cook Time: 12 minutes

Crisp tortilla chips stud this Tex-Mex soup, adding flavor and a crunchy texture. Chili powder is a blend of dried chile (hot) peppers and spices, often garlic, oregano, cumin, and coriander.

	Nonstick cooking spray
1	pound skinless, boneless chicken breasts, chopped
1½	teaspoons chili powder
¾	teaspoon ground cumin
1	14½-ounce can fat-free, low-sodium chicken broth
1	14½-ounce can diced tomatoes with jalapeños, undrained
1½	cups frozen corn
1	cup water
4	green onions, sliced
¼	cup snipped fresh cilantro
¾	cup avocado
3	cups (3 ounces) mini round baked low-sodium tortilla chips, coarsely crushed
1	lime, cut into 4 wedges

1 In large nonstick saucepan lightly sprayed with nonstick cooking spray cook chicken over medium heat for 2 minutes. Add chili powder and cumin; cook, stirring, for 30 seconds.

2 Add broth, tomatoes, corn, and the water; bring to a simmer and cook for 5 minutes. Add green onion; cook for 1 minute. Divide among 4 bowls. Top with cilantro, avocado, and tortilla chips; serve with lime.

Makes 4 servings

COMPLETE MEAL SERVING
441 calories / 12 g total fat / 110 calories from fat / 24% calories from fat
97 mg cholesterol / 900 mg sodium / 43 g carbohydrate / 8 g fiber / 8 g sugars / 43 g protein

moving forward
Take your lunch to work. You'll have more control over what you eat if you prepare it yourself.

Roasted Pepper and Corn Soup

Prep Time: 10 minutes ■ Cook Time: 20 minutes

When selecting chile peppers such as jalapeños, choose ones with an even color and firm texture. The heat comes from the seeds and veins, so be sure to remove and discard them. Wear plastic or rubber gloves while cutting chiles to prevent burns to your fingers.

4	large ears corn, husked and silks removed
	Nonstick cooking spray
1	cup chopped onion (1 large)
2	tablespoons minced jalapeño pepper
2	cups peeled potato cut into ½-inch pieces (2 medium)
1	14-ounce can fat-free, reduced-sodium chicken broth
¼	teaspoon dried thyme, crushed
¾	cup evaporated low-fat milk
1	7-ounce jar roasted red sweet peppers, rinsed, drained, and chopped
6	ounces cooked skinless chicken thighs, shredded

1 Using sharp knife cut away corn kernels from each cob. (You should have about 2 cups corn kernels.)

2 In large saucepan lightly sprayed with nonstick cooking spray cook onion and jalapeño over medium heat for 3 minutes, stirring occasionally. Add corn kernels, potato, broth, thyme, and milk. Increase heat to high; bring mixture to boiling. Reduce heat to low; cover and simmer for 10 minutes. Spoon ¾ cup soup into blender or food processor and blend or process until smooth. Return puree to saucepan with red peppers; heat through. Divide among 4 bowls and top each with chicken.

Makes 4 servings

COMPLETE MEAL SERVING
401 calories / 13 g total fat / 117 calories from fat / 30% calories from fat
42 mg cholesterol / 628 mg sodium / 49 g carbohydrate / 6 g fiber / 9 g sugars / 19 g protein

Chicken and White Bean Chili

Prep Time: 10 minutes ■ Cook Time: 20 minutes

This tomato-less chili is a sure hit for children and adults alike. If your family doesn't like spicy foods, omit the jalapeños.

	Nonstick cooking spray
1	pound skinless, boneless chicken thighs, cut into 1-inch pieces
1	large red sweet pepper, cut into ½-inch pieces
1	cup chopped onion (1 large)
3	tablespoons minced jalapeño pepper (see tip, page 34)
2	cloves garlic, minced
2½	tablespoons all-purpose flour
2¼	cups fat-free, low-sodium chicken broth
1	19-ounce can cannellini beans, rinsed and drained
1	tablespoon ground cumin
2	tablespoons fat-free sour cream
1	cup avocado, diced

1 In large skillet lightly sprayed with nonstick cooking spray cook and stir chicken over medium-high heat for 4 minutes or until brown. With slotted spoon, remove to plate. Lightly spray same skillet with nonstick cooking spray and cook sweet pepper, onion, jalapeño, and garlic, stirring occasionally, for 5 minutes or until light brown and tender.

2 Add flour; cook, stirring, 1 minute. Stir in broth, chicken, beans, and cumin. Bring to boiling over high heat. Reduce heat to low; cover and simmer for 10 minutes or until chicken is no longer pink and vegetables are tender. Remove from heat and stir in sour cream. Garnish with avocado.

Makes 4 servings

to complete the meal For 4 servings: 2 cups cooked quick-cooking brown rice

COMPLETE MEAL SERVING
500 calories / 15 g total fat / 137 calories from fat / 27% calories from fat
95 mg cholesterol / 489 mg sodium / 58 g carbohydrate / 13 g fiber / 6 g sugars / 37 g protein

Chunky Minestrone

Prep Time: 10 minutes ■ Cook Time: 20 minutes

Loaded with vegetables and bits of beef, this hearty soup will satisfy even the hungriest diners. Look for a variety of canned diced tomatoes flavored with everything from balsamic vinegar to mushrooms and try different ones to flavor this soup.

½	cup uncooked orzo
	Nonstick cooking spray
¾	pound lean beef stew meat
3	cloves garlic, minced
1	cup chopped carrot (2 medium)
1	cup chopped onion (1 large)
2	14-ounce cans fat-free, reduced-sodium beef broth
1	14½-ounce can diced tomatoes with basil, garlic, and oregano, undrained
2	cups chopped savoy or green cabbage
1	medium zucchini, halved lengthwise and cut into ¼-inch pieces (1½ cups)
1	15-ounce can small white beans, rinsed and drained
¼	cup grated fat-free Parmesan cheese
½	cup avocado, cubed

1 Prepare orzo according to package directions. Drain.

2 Meanwhile, in large nonstick saucepan lightly sprayed with nonstick cooking spray cook beef, garlic, carrot, and onion over medium-high heat, stirring, for 5 minutes. Add broth, tomatoes, cabbage, and zucchini. Increase heat to high; bring to boiling. Reduce heat to low; cover and simmer for 10 minutes.

3 Stir in orzo and beans; cook for 5 minutes or until vegetables are tender.

4 Divide among 4 bowls; top each bowl with 1 tablespoon cheese and 2 tablespoons avocado.

Makes 4 servings

COMPLETE MEAL SERVING
479 calories / 13 g total fat / 118 calories from fat / 25% calories from fat
51 mg cholesterol / 516 mg sodium / 55 g carbohydrate / 10 g fiber / 11 g sugars / 35 g protein

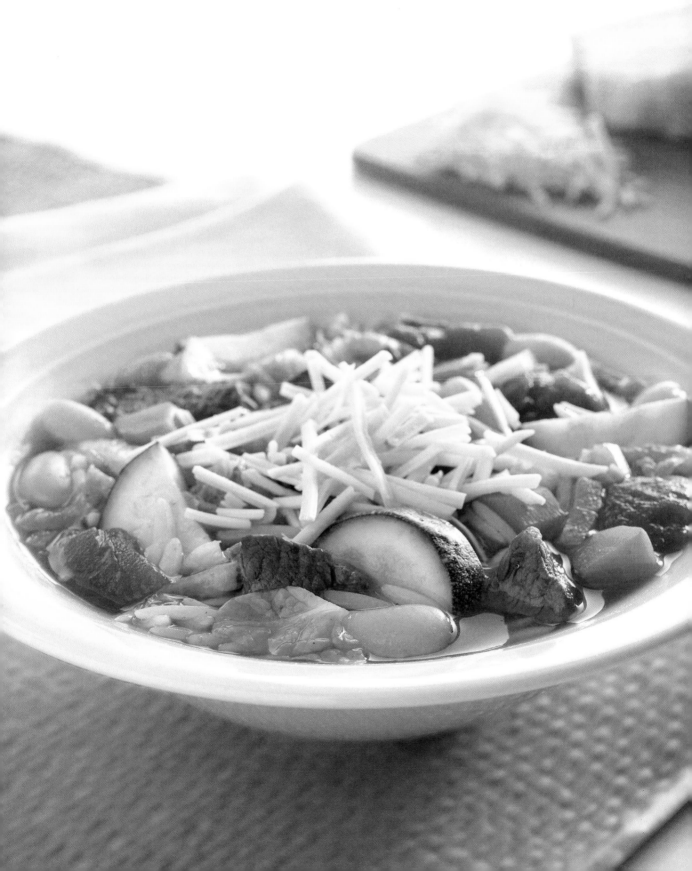

Beef Curry Bowl

Prep Time: 22 minutes ■ Cook Time: 16 minutes

Warm spices—curry, ginger, and cinnamon—season this hearty dish. If you're not fond of eggplant, replace it with an equal amount of yellow squash.

	Nonstick cooking spray
1	pound extra lean ground beef
3	cups cubed peeled eggplant
1½	cups chopped zucchini (1 medium)
2	teaspoons curry powder
¼	teaspoon ground apple pie spice
2	teaspoons chopped fresh ginger
1	14½-ounce can low-sodium beef broth
1	14½-ounce can diced tomatoes with onion and garlic, undrained
1	cup water
1	15-ounce can garbanzo beans, rinsed and drained
½	cup avocado, chopped

1 In large nonstick saucepan lightly sprayed with nonstick cooking spray cook beef over medium-high heat for 5 minutes or until no longer pink. With slotted spoon remove to bowl. Drain any drippings from saucepan. Add eggplant and zucchini to saucepan. Cook, stirring occasionally, for 5 minutes. Stir in curry powder, apple pie spice, and ginger; cook for 30 seconds.

2 Add broth, tomatoes, the water, beans, and beef. Bring to a simmer and cook for 5 minutes or until flavors blend. Garnish with avocado.

Makes 4 servings

to complete the meal   Per serving: one 2½-inch whole wheat roll

COMPLETE MEAL SERVING
394 calories / 12 g total fat / 111 calories from fat / 28% calories from fat
70 mg cholesterol / 849 mg sodium / 39 g carbohydrate / 9 g fiber / 13 g sugars / 34 g protein

Miso Soup with Pork

Prep Time: 20 minutes ■ Cook Time: 20 minutes

Miso, fermented soybean paste, is a staple in Japanese cooking. This thick, salty paste seasons soups and sauces.

6	ounces uncooked udon noodles or whole wheat linguine
	Nonstick cooking spray
12	ounces pork tenderloin, cut into ¼-inch slices
1	14½-ounce can low-sodium chicken broth
2	cups water
2	tablespoons fresh chopped ginger
1	cup firm tofu, cubed
½	pound bok choy or napa (Chinese) cabbage, sliced (stems and leaves kept separate)
1	cup bias-sliced carrot (2 medium)
2	tablespoons white or yellow miso (soybean paste)
¼	cup snipped fresh cilantro

1 Prepare noodles according to package directions; drain.

2 Meanwhile, in large saucepan lightly sprayed with nonstick cooking spray cook pork over medium-high heat for 5 minutes, stirring, until brown and no pink remains. Using slotted spoon, remove pork to bowl. With a paper towel dab any visible drippings from pork. Drain any drippings from saucepan. Add broth, the water, and ginger to saucepan; bring to boiling. Add tofu, bok choy stems, and carrot. Reduce heat to low; simmer for 6 minutes. Stir in miso until dissolved.

3 Add noodles, pork, and bok choy leaves. Cook for 2 minutes or until heated through. Divide among 4 bowls; top with cilantro.

Makes 4 servings

COMPLETE MEAL SERVING
415 calories / 13 g total fat / 116 calories from fat / 27% calories from fat
52 mg cholesterol / 1,246 mg sodium / 40 g carbohydrate / 5 g fiber / 6 g sugars / 37 g protein

Simple Shrimp Paella

Prep Time: 8 minutes ■ Cook Time: 25 minutes

Paella, a Spanish rice dish studded with vegetables, meat, and seafood, usually gets its yellow color from saffron. To avoid the high cost of saffron and add a health boost, this recipe uses turmeric. A powerful antioxidant, turmeric adds only a mild pungency but plenty of color as well as anti-inflammatory and antibacterial benefits.

	Nonstick cooking spray
4	ounces spicy turkey sausage, casing removed, crumbled
1	cup uncooked long grain white rice
2	cups fat-free, low-sodium chicken broth
½	tablespoon mild hot sauce (or to taste)
¼	teaspoon ground turmeric
1	pound peeled and deveined medium shrimp
1	medium tomato, chopped
1	cup frozen green peas
½	cup sliced green onion
⅓	cup sliced black olives

1 In medium saucepan lightly sprayed with nonstick cooking spray cook sausage over medium heat for 5 minutes, stirring, until brown. With slotted spoon remove to bowl. With paper towel dab sausage to remove any visible drippings. Add rice, broth, hot sauce, and turmeric to same saucepan; bring to boiling. Reduce heat to low; cover and simmer for 15 minutes or until most of the broth is absorbed.

2 Stir in shrimp, tomato, peas, green onion, and olives; cover and simmer for 5 minutes or until the rice is tender and shrimp are opaque. Stir in sausage. Heat through.

Makes 4 servings

COMPLETE MEAL SERVING
461 calories / 14 g total fat / 122 calories from fat / 27% calories from fat
193 mg cholesterol / 968 mg sodium / 49 g carbohydrate / 4 g fiber / 35 g sugars / 41 g protein

Salmon Posole

Prep Time: 5 minutes ■ Cook Time: 20 minutes

Posole, a traditional Mexican soup, features hominy, onion, garlic, chile peppers, and pork. Here healthful salmon replaces the pork. Hominy is corn kernels that have been dried with the hull and germ removed. (Ground hominy is called grits.) The kernels become reconstituted when canned, making them ready to eat.

2   8-inch corn tortillas, cut into ½-inch strips
     Nonstick cooking spray
1   cup chopped onion (1 large)
2   tablespoons minced garlic
2   tablespoons minced jalapeño pepper (see tip, page 34)
½   teaspoon dried oregano, crushed
3   cups white hominy, rinsed and drained
2   14½-ounce cans no-salt-added stewed tomatoes, undrained
2   cups water
2   7½-ounce cans red salmon, skin and bones removed, broken into 1-inch pieces
4   green onions, sliced
2   teaspoons grated lime zest
3   tablespoons low-sodium, low-fat cheddar cheese
3   tablespoons sour cream

1 Preheat oven to 425°F.

2 Place tortillas on baking sheet and lightly spray with nonstick cooking spray. Bake, turning once, for 5 minutes or until lightly brown. Remove to rack to cool.

3 In large saucepan lightly sprayed with nonstick cooking spray cook onion, garlic, jalapeño, and oregano over medium-high heat for 5 minutes, stirring occasionally. Add hominy, tomatoes, and the water. Bring to boiling over high heat. Reduce heat to low; simmer for 10 minutes or until onion is tender. Stir in salmon, green onion, and zest; heat through.

4 Divide soup among 4 bowls. Divide tortilla strips among bowls and serve in soup. Garnish with cheese and sour cream.

Makes 4 servings

COMPLETE MEAL SERVING
433 calories / 12 g total fat / 109 calories from fat / 25% calories from fat
87 mg cholesterol / 848 mg sodium / 46 g carbohydrate / 9 g fiber / 16 g sugars / 39 g protein

Tortellini Squash Soup

Prep Time: 5 minutes ■ Cook Time: 20 minutes

To vary the seasonings of this soup, add a pinch of cinnamon just before serving. It will complement the caramel-roasted flavor of the squash. Or if you prefer, use a sprinkling of chopped cilantro to add brightness to the whole dish, or ginger and nutmeg to add warmth.

1	medium buttercup squash (2½ to 3 pounds), halved lengthwise
2	9-ounce packages fresh whole wheat tortellini with three cheeses
2	cups low-sodium chicken broth
2	cups water
¼	teaspoon ground black pepper

1 Place 1 sheet of microwave-safe plastic wrap on the floor of microwave and place squash halves, cut sides down, on the plastic. Microwave on 100% power (high) for 15 minutes or until squash is cooked through.

2 Meanwhile, in large saucepan prepare tortellini according to package directions. Drain and set aside. In same saucepan bring broth, the water, and pepper to a simmer over medium heat.

3 When squash is cool enough to handle, scoop out and discard squash seeds and "strings." Scrape squash meat directly into food processor or blender. Add 2 cups of the broth mixture and process or blend until smooth. Return to saucepan with remaining broth mixture. Stir in tortellini. Cook for 5 minutes or until heated through.

Makes 6 servings

COMPLETE MEAL SERVING
391 calories / 12 g total fat / 113 calories from fat / 29% calories from fat
54 mg cholesterol / 611 mg sodium / 52 g carbohydrate / 10 g fiber / 6 g sugars / 19 g protein

moving forward
Sneak in some extra activity whenever you can, such as taking a walk around the mall before shopping.

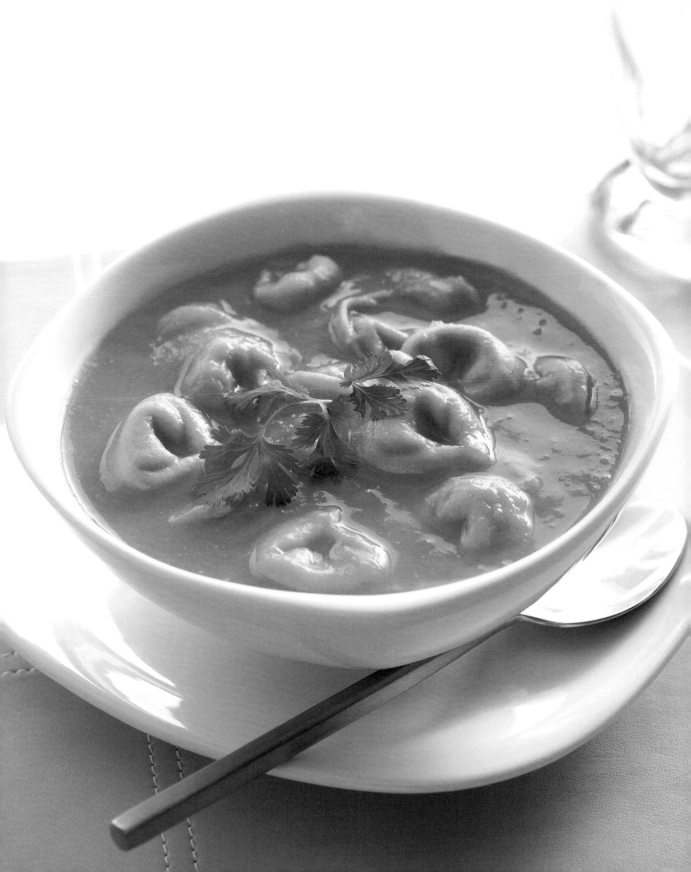

Tropical Chicken Salad

Prep Time: 15 minutes

When you're in the mood for Thai takeout, this dish is the perfect way to satisfy your craving. The cilantro is cool and refreshing, making this dish the right choice for hot summer days and easy entertaining.

4	cups baby spinach
2	cups loosely packed cilantro leaves
3	cups shredded cooked chicken breast (about 12 ounces)
1½	cups cooked brown rice
1	red sweet pepper, very thinly sliced
1	mango, peeled, seeded, and cut into ½-inch chunks
1	cup blueberries
½	red onion, very thinly sliced
½	cup fat-free honey dijon salad dressing
½	cup dry-roasted unsalted cashews

In large bowl combine spinach, cilantro, chicken, rice, sweet pepper, mango, blueberries, and onion. Drizzle with salad dressing and sprinkle with cashews. Toss to coat well.

Makes 4 servings

COMPLETE MEAL SERVING
426 calories / 12 g total fat / 110 calories from fat / 25% calories from fat
35 mg cholesterol / 678 mg sodium / 59 g carbohydrate / 10 g fiber / 19 g sugars / 22 g protein

Tabbouleh with Chicken

Prep Time: 30 minutes

Bulgur, the main ingredient in any tabbouleh, is whole wheat kernels that have been boiled, dried, and cracked. Bulgur has an earthy flavor and a tender but chewy texture, and it is a staple in Middle Eastern dishes.

1¼	cups boiling water
1	cup uncooked bulgur
⅓	cup lemon juice
½	teaspoon salt (optional)
¼	teaspoon ground black pepper
12	ounces cooked skinless, boneless chicken breast, thinly sliced
2	cups seeded and chopped tomatoes
½	cup raisins
½	cup chopped green onion (4)
½	cup snipped fresh parsley
¼	cup snipped fresh mint
½	cup shredded cheddar cheese
¼	cup feta cheese

1 In large bowl pour the boiling water over bulgur; let stand for 30 minutes.

2 Meanwhile, in large serving bowl whisk together lemon juice, salt (if desired), and pepper. Add chicken, tomato, raisins, green onion, parsley, and mint. Toss to coat well.

3 Add bulgur and cheeses; toss well.

Makes 4 servings

COMPLETE MEAL SERVING
425 calories / 13 g total fat / 119 calories from fat / 27% calories from fat
63 mg cholesterol / 874 mg sodium / 54 g carbohydrate / 9 g fiber / 16 g sugars / 26 g protein

Chinese Chicken Salad

Prep Time: 20 minutes ■ Cook Time: 6 minutes

Hoisin sauce, sometimes called Peking sauce, is a thick brown sauce with a sweet and sour flavor that is commonly used in Chinese cooking. Look for the blend of soybeans, garlic, hot peppers, sugar, and vinegar in the ethnic section of the supermarket.

1	pound skinless, boneless chicken breasts, thinly sliced
2	tablespoons low-sodium soy sauce
2	tablespoons minced fresh ginger, divided
⅓	cup hoisin sauce
⅓	cup orange marmalade fruit spread
3	tablespoons seasoned rice wine vinegar
2	tablespoons water
4	cups sliced napa cabbage
1	red sweet pepper, cut into ¼-inch strips
1	cup cucumber, partially peeled, cut lengthwise in half, then sliced
1	cup shredded carrot (2 medium)
	Nonstick cooking spray
¼	cup raw cashews, chopped

1 Place chicken in resealable plastic bag with soy sauce and 2 teaspoons of the ginger. Turn bag over several times to coat chicken with dressing; set aside.

2 Meanwhile, in large bowl whisk together hoisin sauce, marmalade, vinegar, the water, and the remaining 1 tablespoon plus 1 teaspoon ginger. Add cabbage, sweet pepper, cucumber, and carrot. Toss to coat well.

3 Drain chicken; discard marinade. In large skillet lightly sprayed with nonstick cooking spray cook chicken over medium heat, turning, for 6 minutes or until no longer pink. Add to salad and toss. Garnish with cashews.

Makes 4 servings

COMPLETE MEAL SERVING
331 calories / 11 g total fat / 100 calories from fat / 30% calories from fat
48 mg cholesterol / 1,109 mg sodium / 37 g carbohydrate / 4 g fiber / 19 g sugars / 22 g protein

Chicken with Fruit and Fennel Salad

Prep Time: 15 minutes

Ready in minutes, this flavorful salad is bursting with nutrients. Fresh fruit and vegetables blended with chunks of chicken make this dish an antioxidant-rich meal.

- ¼ cup lime juice
- ¼ teaspoon salt (optional)
- ¼ teaspoon cracked black pepper
- 1 pound skinless, boneless chicken breasts, cooked and cut into 1-inch pieces
- 3 large nectarines, peeled, pitted, and sliced
- 1 cup blueberries
- 1 medium head fennel, cored and very thinly sliced
- 1 cup loosely packed fresh cilantro, roughly chopped
- ½ medium red onion, very thinly sliced
- 3 tablespoons chopped avocado
- 3 tablespoons dry roasted, unsalted pecans

In large bowl whisk together lime juice, salt (if desired), and pepper. Add chicken, nectarines, blueberries, fennel, cilantro, onion, avocado, and pecans. Toss to coat well.

Makes 4 servings

COMPLETE MEAL SERVING
355 calories / 12 g total fat / 105 calories from fat / 29% calories from fat
96 mg cholesterol / 129 mg sodium / 26 g carbohydrate / 7 g fiber / 13 g sugars / 39 g protein

moving forward
Keep a food journal. Writing down everything you eat has been proven to keep dieters on track and honest.

Mesclun Salad with Turkey, Pears, and Cherries

Prep Time: 15 minutes

This tart-sweet salad makes a lovely lunch after the holidays. Toss cooked turkey and greens with a combination of fruits and nuts for a surprisingly delicious meal.

½	cup fat-free cranberry-walnut vinaigrette
2	tablespoons orange marmalade fruit spread
8	cups mesclun
12	ounces skinless, cooked turkey breast, cut into ¾-inch cubes
1	red Bartlett pear, cut into ¼-inch slices
½	medium red onion, thinly sliced
½	cup dried cherries
⅓	cup toasted hazelnuts, dried, roasted, no salt, coarsely chopped

1 In small bowl whisk together vinaigrette and marmalade.

2 Arrange mesclun on large platter. Top with turkey, pear, onion, cherries, and hazelnuts. Drizzle with dressing and toss to coat.

Makes 4 servings

COMPLETE MEAL SERVING
361 calories / 12 g total fat / 109 calories from fat / 29% calories from fat
71 mg cholesterol / 362 mg sodium / 37 g carbohydrate / 7 g fiber / 25 g sugars / 30 g protein

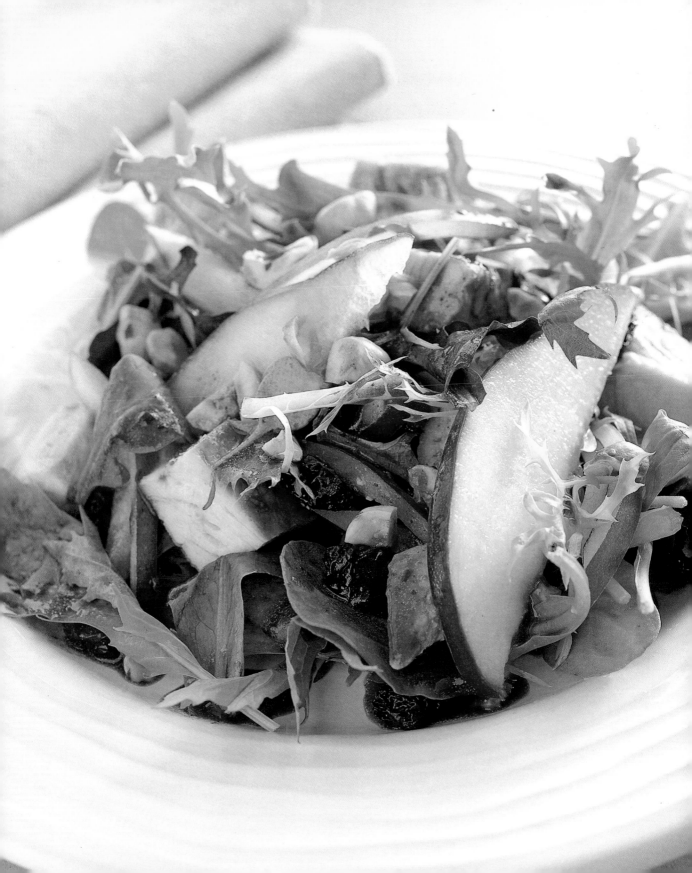

Chesapeake Chicken Salad

Prep Time: 5 minutes ■ Cook Time: 5 minutes

Old Bay seasoning and crabmeat add the flavors of the Chesapeake Bay to ordinary chicken breasts. When grilling chicken breasts for dinner, throw four extra ones on the grill and refrigerate for the next day. You'll be ready to prepare this spectacular dish in just minutes.

½   cup imitation crabmeat
1   tablespoon chopped yellow sweet pepper
1   tablespoon chopped red sweet pepper
1   teaspoon Old Bay seasoning
1   cup low-fat plain yogurt
4   grilled skinless, boneless chicken breasts (1 pound)
4   cups salad greens
⅓   cup fat-free balsamic vinaigrette
⅓   cup shredded low-fat cheddar cheese
1¼   cups avocado, diced

1 Preheat oven to 350°F.

2 In medium bowl combine crab, sweet peppers, seasoning, and yogurt.

3 Place chicken on cutting board. With sharp knife parallel to surface, cut 1 chicken breast in half lengthwise. Repeat with remaining chicken breasts.

4 Place bottom halves of the chicken breasts on baking sheet. Divide crab mixture over chicken. Top with top halves of the chicken breasts. Bake for 5 minutes or until hot.

5 Meanwhile, place greens on large platter. Drizzle with vinaigrette and sprinkle with cheese and avocado; toss to coat. Top with chicken.

Makes 4 servings

to complete the meal   Per serving: one 2½-inch whole wheat dinner roll

COMPLETE MEAL SERVING
307 calories / 11 g total fat / 94 calories from fat / 31% calories from fat
73 mg cholesterol / 692 mg sodium / 18 g carbohydrate / 5 g fiber / 7 g sugars / 34 g protein

Taco Salad

Prep Time: 15 minutes

Satisfy a hungry crowd with this hearty, flavorful meal. It's perfect for parties, tailgates, or simple lunches at home.

½	cup fat-free ranch dressing
¼	cup chunky salsa
2	tablespoons snipped fresh cilantro
8	cups torn romaine lettuce
1	large tomato, seeded and chopped
8	ounces lean roast beef, shredded (2 cups)
1	15-ounce can black beans, rinsed and drained
1½	cups corn kernels, fresh or frozen and thawed
4	ounces shredded low-fat Monterey Jack cheese (1 cup)
½	cup coarsely chopped green onion (4)
1	6¾-ounce bag baked tortilla chips
½	cup avocado, diced

In large bowl whisk together dressing, salsa, and cilantro. Add lettuce, tomato, beef, beans, corn, cheese, and green onion; toss to coat. Place tortilla chips on large serving platter. Top with salad. Garnish with avocado.

Makes 6 servings

COMPLETE MEAL SERVING
427 calories / 13 g total fat / 113 calories from fat / 26% calories from fat
50 mg cholesterol / 735 mg sodium / 54 g carbohydrate / 8 g fiber / 5 g sugars / 28 g protein

---

moving forward

Give yourself reminders to take your alli capsule—leave the capsules where you'll see them or take the carrying case with you wherever you go.

Chopped Greek Salad with Steak

Prep Time: 15 minutes

Refreshing and flavorful, this main dish salad is perfect for hot summer days. Using leftover steak makes the meal ready in minutes. If you don't have leftover steak, grill or broil a lean steak such as flank or top round while making the salad. The salad will still be ready in less than 20 minutes.

6	cups torn romaine lettuce
2	tablespoons snipped fresh mint
2	tablespoons snipped fresh dillweed
2	cups grape tomatoes, halved
1	cup chopped cucumber (½ medium)
1	cup canned garbanzo beans, rinsed and drained
⅓	cup coarsely chopped kalamata olives
½	cup fat-free Italian dressing
8	ounces lean cooked steak, thinly sliced
2	tablespoons reduced-fat crumbled feta cheese
½	medium avocado, peeled, pitted, and chopped
¼	cup pine nuts

1 In large bowl combine lettuce, mint, dillweed, tomatoes, cucumber, beans, olives, and dressing, tossing to coat well.

2 Divide among 4 salad plates. Top each with one-fourth of the steak. Divide cheese, avocado, and pine nuts over each plate.

Makes 4 servings

to complete the meal   Per serving: one 4-inch whole wheat pita

COMPLETE MEAL SERVING
332 calories / 12 g total fat / 105 calories from fat / 30% calories from fat
35 mg cholesterol / 791 mg sodium / 36 g carbohydrate / 8 g fiber / 3 g sugars / 24 g protein

Quinoa, Veggie, and Pork Toss

Prep Time: 20 minutes ■ Cook Time: 17 minutes

This tasty salad is perfect to pack for picnics or brown-bagged lunches because it can be refrigerated for up to one day in advance.

¾	cup uncooked quinoa
1½	cups water
½	teaspoon salt (optional)
1	cup frozen corn
1	cup frozen sugar snap peas
1	cup chopped red sweet pepper (1 large)
1	pound cooked pork tenderloin, cut into 1-inch pieces
¼	cup chopped green onion (2)
¼	cup fat-free lime vinaigrette
½	cup green olives, sliced
5	tablespoons walnuts, chopped

1 Place quinoa in sieve and rinse well under cold running water.

2 In medium saucepan combine quinoa, the water, and salt (if desired). Bring to a simmer; cover and cook for 12 minutes.

3 Stir in corn and peas. Return to simmer and cook for 5 minutes or until quinoa is tender and liquid is absorbed. Place quinoa mixture in medium bowl; stir in sweet pepper, pork, green onion, vinaigrette, olives, and walnuts.

Makes 4 servings

COMPLETE MEAL SERVING
362 calories / 12 g total fat / 109 calories from fat / 29% calories from fat
49 mg cholesterol / 633 mg sodium / 38 g carbohydrate / 5 g fiber / 5 g sugars / 28 g protein

moving forward
Each day you stay on the alli weight loss plan you are one day closer to your weight goal.

Winter Salad Delight

Prep Time: 10 minutes ■ Cook Time: 20 minutes

Healthy soul food at its best is how one would describe this dish. Hearty greens—kale, mustard, and spinach—are sauteed and tossed with a syrupy dressing and then topped with spicy cooked shrimp.

Dressing	2	tablespoons apple cider vinegar
	2	tablespoons balsamic vinegar
Salad	1½	pounds kale
	1½	pounds mustard greens
	2	slices 100% stone-ground wheat bread
	1	pound peeled and deveined large shrimp
	¼	teaspoon salt (optional)
	¼	teaspoon crushed red pepper flakes
		Nonstick cooking spray
	2	tablespoons water
	1	10-ounce bag spinach
	1	cup avocado, chopped

1 For dressing, in small saucepan combine apple cider vinegar and balsamic vinegar over medium-high heat. Bring to boiling and boil for 5 minutes or until syrupy.

2 Meanwhile, wash kale thoroughly in cold water; drain well. Remove and discard stems. Coarsely chop leaves to measure 6 cups; set aside. Repeat with mustard greens.

3 Toast bread; cut into 1-inch pieces; set aside.

4 For salad, season shrimp with salt (if desired) and red pepper flakes.

5 In large nonstick skillet lightly sprayed with nonstick cooking spray cook shrimp over medium heat, turning, for 5 minutes or until opaque. Remove to plate. Add kale and cook, turning with tongs, for 2 minutes or until kale starts to wilt. Add mustard greens; cook, turning with tongs, for 6 minutes or until wilted. Add the water, cover, and cook for 5 minutes or until tender. Add spinach and dressing; cook for 2 minutes.

6 Place greens in large bowl and top with shrimp. Top with toasted bread cubes and avocado.

Makes 4 servings

COMPLETE MEAL SERVING
402 calories / 13 g total fat / 116 calories from fat / 27% calories from fat
172 mg cholesterol / 455 mg sodium / 41 g carbohydrate / 15 g fiber / 9 g sugars / 37 g protein

Pesto Pasta Salad with Shrimp

Prep Time: 10 minutes ■ Cook Time: 10 minutes

Cavatappi means "corkscrew" in Italian, although this pasta is really more "S" shape and often hollow. You can substitute rotelle, fusilli, or campanelle for the cavatappi in this dish.

8	ounces uncooked cavatappi pasta
1	large potato (12 ounces), peeled and cut into 1-inch cubes
8	ounces green beans, trimmed and halved
¾	pound peeled, deveined, and halved extra-large shrimp
½	cup fresh basil, chopped
1	pint red and/or yellow grape tomatoes, halved
½	cup pine nuts

1 Bring large pot water to boiling. Add pasta; cook for 10 minutes. Add potato 5 minutes before end of pasta cooking time; add green beans 2 minutes before end of pasta cooking time; add shrimp 1 minute before end of pasta cooking time. Reserve ¼ cup pasta water; drain pasta, vegetables, and shrimp.

2 In large bowl fold basil with reserved pasta water. Add pasta mixture and tomatoes. Toss to coat well. Garnish with pine nuts.

Makes 4 servings

COMPLETE MEAL SERVING
518 calories / 14 g total fat / 129 calories from fat / 25% calories from fat
129 mg cholesterol / 138 mg sodium / 69 g carbohydrate / 5 g fiber / 4 g sugars / 30 g protein

moving forward

Take more time to eat and it will help you to realize when you're full. What's the rush? Slow down. Try to stretch a meal by taking small bites and putting your fork down in between.

Herbed Tuna and White Bean Salad

Prep Time: 15 minutes ■ Cook Time: 13 minutes

Here lemon juice and rosemary spice up bottled salad dressing, but if you're short on time, use the salad dressing as it is.

⅔	cup fat-free sundried tomato Italian dressing
3	tablespoons lemon juice
2	tablespoons snipped fresh rosemary
1	pound fresh or frozen tuna steaks
	Nonstick cooking spray
2	cups chopped fennel (1 stalk)
1	cup chopped red onion (1 large)
2	15-ounce cans small white beans, rinsed and drained
2	cups (1 pint) grape tomatoes, halved
4	cups baby arugula
1	cup sliced green olives
½	cup pine nuts

1 In small bowl combine dressing, lemon juice, and rosemary. Remove ⅓ cup of the dressing mixture and place in resealable plastic bag. Add tuna; seal bag and turn to coat. Marinate for 15 minutes, turning occasionally.

2 Meanwhile, in large nonstick skillet lightly sprayed with nonstick cooking spray cook fennel and onion over medium heat for 5 minutes or until crisp-tender. Add beans and remove from heat. Add tomatoes and remaining dressing mixture. Line serving plate with arugula; top with bean mixture.

3 In same skillet cook tuna over medium-high heat, turning once, for 8 minutes or until fish begins to flake when tested with fork. Slice tuna and place on top of bean mixture. Garnish with olives and pine nuts.

Makes 6 servings

COMPLETE MEAL SERVING
367 calories / 13 g total fat / 88 calories from fat / 30% calories from fat
29 mg cholesterol / 354 mg sodium / 36 g carbohydrate / 8 g fiber / 6 g sugars / 29 g protein

Cobb Salad with Salmon

Prep Time: 20 minutes ■ Cook Time: 13 minutes

Canadian bacon, called back bacon north of the border, is more like ham than bacon. This low-fat meat is a healthy substitute for bacon. Like ham, it's fully cooked so it needs cooking only to brown and warm.

2	oranges
⅓	cup fat-free red wine vinegar salad dressing
½	cup sliced green onion
½	cup orange marmalade fruit spread
½	pound wild salmon fillets
3	1-ounce slices Canadian bacon
1	5-ounce package baby arugula
2	tomatoes, cored and sliced
½	cup avocado
2	large hard-cooked eggs, peeled, halved, yolk discarded, and whites chopped

1 Preheat broiler.

2 Meanwhile, grate enough orange zest to measure 1 teaspoon. Remove peel and pith from oranges. Working over bowl to catch any juices, cut oranges into segments. Squeeze orange membranes to extract any remaining juice. Set oranges aside.

3 Place dressing in medium bowl. Whisk 2 tablespoons orange juice into dressing.

4 In another medium bowl stir 2 tablespoons orange juice, zest, and 3 tablespoons of the green onion into marmalade.

5 Arrange salmon on rack in broiler pan. Broil salmon 6 inches from heat for 8 minutes. Brush salmon with marmalade mixture and continue cooking for 5 minutes or until salmon is opaque.

6 While salmon cooks heat bacon in nonstick skillet over medium heat for 2 minutes, turning once. Drain on paper towels. Slice bacon into thin strips.

7 Place arugula on serving plate. Arrange tomato slices, avocado, orange sections, and salmon on plate. Sprinkle with bacon, egg white, and remaining green onion. Serve with dressing.

Makes 4 servings

COMPLETE MEAL SERVING
350 calories / 12 g total fat / 109 calories from fat / 29% calories from fat
148 mg cholesterol / 345 mg sodium / 43 g carbohydrate / 6 g fiber / 34 g sugars / 22 g protein

Sensational Salmon Salad

Prep Time: 10 minutes

Adding cranberries to salads is a delicious idea, and a healthy one too. Cousin to blueberries, this native American berry contains beneficial antioxidants as well as vitamins C and K, and it's a very good source of fiber.

4½	cups torn romaine lettuce
3	ripe apples, thinly sliced
⅓	cup dried cranberries
⅓	cup sliced almonds
½	cup shredded Parmesan cheese
½	cup fat-free creamy Italian dressing
⅔	cup part-skim ricotta cheese
2	6-ounce pouches salmon fillets, drained and patted dry

In large bowl combine lettuce, apple slices, cranberries, almonds, and cheese. Drizzle with dressing, tossing to coat. Divide salad and ricotta cheese among 4 plates. Divide salmon among plates.

Makes 4 servings

to complete the meal   Per serving: 2 plain crisp 7-inch breadsticks

COMPLETE MEAL SERVING
310 calories / 11 g total fat / 100 calories from fat / 30% calories from fat
138 mg cholesterol / 593 mg sodium / 38 g carbohydrate / 5 g fiber / 23 g sugars / 20 g protein

moving forward

Make a habit of reading nutrition labels before you buy packaged foods. It will help you make smart choices.

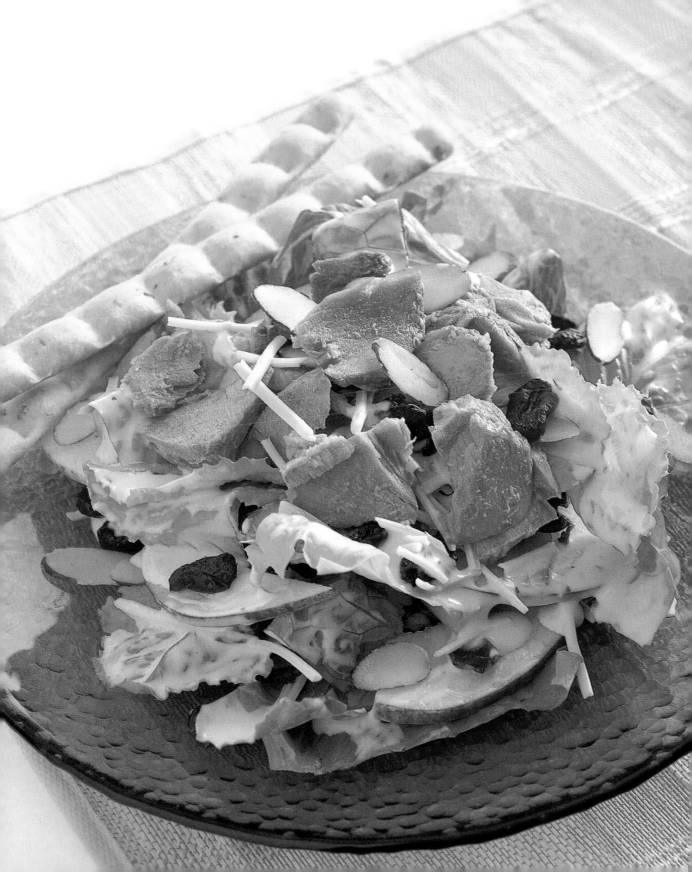

Gazpacho Salad with Goat Cheese

Prep Time: 12 minutes

Seedless cucumbers, also known as English or burpless cucumbers, actually do contain seeds. However, they are so small they don't need to be removed. Look for long, thin seedless cucumbers wrapped in plastic.

8	ounces uncooked whole wheat shell or penne pasta
2	tablespoons red wine vinegar
½	teaspoon hot sauce
¼	to ½ teaspoon salt (optional)
1	pound vine-ripened tomatoes (4 medium), diced
1½	cups chopped seedless cucumber (1 medium)
1½	cups chopped yellow sweet pepper (2 large)
4	radishes, sliced in quarter rounds (¾ cup)
½	cup fresh basil leaves, cut into thin slivers
6	ounces reduced-fat goat cheese, crumbled

1 Prepare pasta according to package directions. Drain.

2 Meanwhile, in large bowl whisk together vinegar, hot sauce, and salt (if desired) until blended. Toss in tomato, cucumber, sweet pepper, radishes, and pasta until combined.

3 Toss in half of the basil just until combined. Place salad in 4 bowls. Divide cheese over bowls and sprinkle each with remaining basil.

Makes 4 servings

COMPLETE MEAL SERVING
402 calories / 14 g total fat / 125 calories from fat / 30% calories from fat
34 mg cholesterol / 390 mg sodium / 51 g carbohydrate / 4 g fiber / 7 g sugars / 21 g protein

Tomato, Basil, and Mozzarella Pasta Salad

Prep Time: 20 minutes ■ Cook Time: 8 minutes

The fresh flavors of summer highlight this Italian-inspired salad. In the dead of winter, substitute 1¼ pounds of vine-ripened cherry tomatoes for the tomatoes.

2	cups uncooked whole wheat farfalle or orecchiette pasta
⅓	cup chopped dried tomatoes
1¼	pounds tomatoes, chopped (2 cups)
2	tablespoons red wine vinegar
1	shallot, halved
¼	teaspoon ground black pepper
4	ounces fresh mozzarella cheese, cubed (¾ cup)
¾	cup fresh basil leaves, torn

1 Prepare pasta according to package directions. Rinse in colander under cold running water; drain well.

2 Meanwhile, remove ½ cup boiling water from pasta saucepan and combine with dried tomatoes in small bowl; set aside for 5 minutes.

3 In blender combine 1 cup of the chopped tomato, vinegar, shallot, and pepper; blend until smooth.

4 In large bowl combine remaining 1 cup tomato and cheese.

5 Drain dried tomatoes and add to bowl with basil, pasta, and blended tomato dressing; toss to coat well.

Makes 2 servings

COMPLETE MEAL SERVING
397 calories / 13 g total fat / 116 calories from fat / 27% calories from fat
31 mg cholesterol / 506 mg sodium / 48 g carbohydrate / 6 g fiber / 13 g sugars / 31 g protein

Summer Tostada Salad

Prep Time: 15 minutes ■ Cook Time: 5 minutes

Bursting with fresh flavors, these tostadas are sure to please. A fresh tomato salad tops corn tortillas layered with lettuce, beans, cheese, and avocado.

3	medium tomatoes, chopped
¼	cup snipped fresh cilantro
¼	cup chopped red onion
2	tablespoons lime juice
1	tablespoon mild hot sauce (or to taste)
8	6-inch corn tortillas
6	romaine lettuce leaves, finely shredded
1	15-ounce can black beans, rinsed and drained
¾	cup shredded low-fat mozzarella cheese
1	medium avocado, halved, pitted, peeled, and sliced

1 Preheat oven to 350°F.

2 In medium bowl combine tomato, cilantro, onion, lime juice, and hot sauce. Set aside.

3 Place tortillas on baking sheet and bake for 5 minutes or until crispy and golden.

4 To serve, place 2 tortillas on each of 4 large plates. Divide lettuce, beans, cheese, and avocado evenly over tortillas. Divide tomato mixture over each.

Makes 4 servings

COMPLETE MEAL SERVING
423 calories / 14 g total fat / 127 calories from fat / 30% calories from fat
15 mg cholesterol / 427 mg sodium / 53 g carbohydrate / 14 g fiber / 5 g sugars / 23 g protein

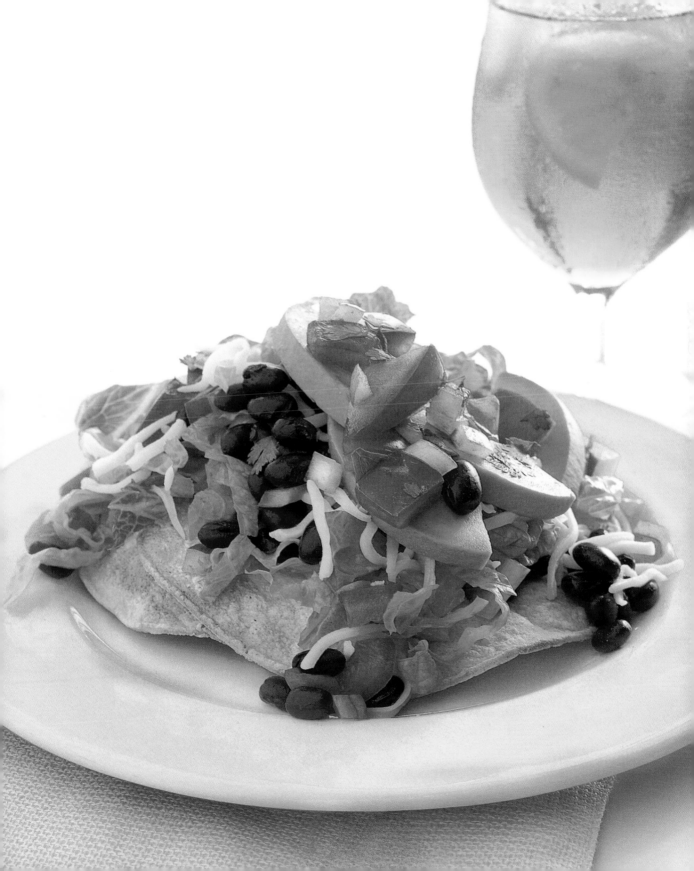

Black-Eyed Pea Salad

Prep Time: 10 minutes

Nothing captures the sense of soul food like black-eyed peas. A seasonal vegetable in the South, black-eyed peas are ingredients in many Southern dishes. Thanks to canning, they are available year-round.

2	tablespoons cider vinegar
2	tablespoons honey
2	cloves garlic, minced
¼	teaspoon salt (optional)
¼	teaspoon ground black pepper
2	15-ounce cans black-eyed peas, rinsed and drained
10	ounces firm baked tofu, cut into ¼-inch pieces
1	cup chopped red sweet pepper (1)
1	cup chopped green sweet pepper (1)
1	cup chopped celery (2 stalks)
½	cup chopped onion
½	cup raw peanuts, chopped

In large bowl whisk together vinegar, honey, garlic, salt (if desired), and black pepper. Add peas, tofu, sweet peppers, celery, and onion. Toss to coat well. Sprinkle peanuts on top.

Makes 4 servings

to complete the meal   For 4 servings: two 6½-inch whole wheat pitas, halved

COMPLETE MEAL SERVING
430 calories / 14 g total fat / 127 calories from fat / 28% calories from fat
0 mg cholesterol / 692 mg sodium / 60 g carbohydrate / 15 g fiber / 15 g sugars / 24 g protein

Sausage and Pepper Sandwiches

Prep Time: 5 minutes ■ Cook Time: 16 minutes

Hearty and delicious, this classic Italian combination is made healthier with turkey sausage. The fennel seeds impart a characteristic anise flavor, but feel free to omit.

Nonstick cooking spray

12 ounces lean hot Italian turkey sausage, cut into ½-inch slices

1 sweet onion, sliced

3 cups frozen mixed sweet peppers

¼ teaspoon ground black pepper

¼ teaspoon crushed fennel seeds (optional)

1 tablespoon balsamic vinegar

4 3-ounce whole grain rolls, split

½ cup black olives, sliced

1 In a large nonstick skillet lightly sprayed with nonstick cooking spray cook and stir sausage for 5 minutes over medium-high heat or until brown. Remove to bowl with slotted spoon. With a paper towel dab sausage to remove any drippings.

2 In the skillet cook onion for 5 minutes over medium-high heat, stirring occasionally. Stir in sausage, frozen sweet peppers, black pepper, and fennel seeds (if desired). Cover and cook for 5 minutes or until vegetables are tender.

3 Increase heat to high. Stir in vinegar and cook for 1 minute or until liquid is almost evaporated. Place 1 roll on each of 4 plates. Divide sausage mixture among rolls. Garnish with olives.

Makes 4 servings

COMPLETE MEAL SERVING
414 calories / 14 g total fat / 123 calories from fat / 28% calories from fat
42 mg cholesterol / 1,218 mg sodium / 56 g carbohydrate / 9 g fiber / 13 g sugars / 22 g protein

moving forward

Brush your teeth after each meal. Your minty fresh mouth will say "No more food."

Canadian BLTs

Prep Time: 10 minutes ■ Cook Time: 3 minutes

Jarlsberg cheese hails from Norway and is a mild Emmentaler-style cheese with a nutty flavor and buttery texture. An all-purpose cheese, it's good for cooking and for eating out of hand as a snack.

1½	tablespoons reduced-fat mayonnaise
1	clove garlic, minced
1	tablespoon lemon juice
	Nonstick cooking spray
1	6-ounce package sliced Canadian bacon
4	cups packed baby spinach leaves
8	slices multigrain bread, toasted
3	ounces low-sodium mozzarella cheese, sliced
1	tomato, sliced
½	cup sliced avocado

1 In small bowl combine mayonnaise, garlic, and lemon juice until blended; set aside.

2 In large nonstick skillet lightly sprayed with nonstick cooking spray cook bacon over medium-high heat for 2 minutes or until brown, turning once. Remove to plate and pat with paper towel to absorb fat. Add spinach to skillet and cook, stirring frequently, for 1 minute or just until wilted.

3 Place 1 slice bread on each of 4 plates; spread each with 1 tablespoon of the mayonnaise mixture. Divide bacon, cheese, spinach, and tomato on mayonnaise. Top each with 1 slice avocado and bread.

Makes 4 servings

COMPLETE MEAL SERVING
366 calories / 12 g total fat / 108 calories from fat / 28% calories from fat
34 mg cholesterol / 1,098 mg sodium / 45 g carbohydrate / 6 g fiber / 10 g sugars / 24 g protein

Curried Chicken Salad Sandwiches

Prep Time: 15 minutes

Chutney, an Indian condiment, gets its name from the Hindu word chatni, *meaning "strongly spiced." A blend of fruits, vinegar, sugar, and spices, chutney is available in a range of textures, chunky to smooth, and spice levels, hot to mild.*

12	ounces cooked chicken breast, shredded (3 cups)
½	Gala apple, cut into ½-inch pieces (1 cup)
3	tablespoons chopped walnuts
¼	cup chopped green onion (2)
1	tablespoon reduced-fat mayonnaise
½	cup plain low-fat yogurt
2	tablespoons mango chutney
¼	teaspoon curry powder
8	slices whole grain bread

In large bowl combine chicken, apple, walnuts, green onion, mayonnaise, yogurt, chutney, and curry powder. Evenly divide among 4 slices of bread. Top with remaining bread slices.

Makes 4 servings

COMPLETE MEAL SERVING
358 calories / 12 g total fat / 110 calories from fat / 27% calories from fat
45 mg cholesterol / 729 mg sodium / 50 g carbohydrate / 8 g fiber / 13 g sugars / 23 g protein

moving forward

Take a seat. Eating your meals seated at a table focuses your attention on the activity of eating.

Roasted Red Pepper and Chicken Panini

Prep Time: 15 minutes ■ Cook Time: 16 minutes

Broiling your own red sweet peppers adds a delicious smoky flavor to these sandwiches. When time is short, eliminate step 1 and substitute one 7-ounce jar roasted red peppers.

2 red sweet peppers, halved and seeded
    Nonstick cooking spray
1 pound skinless, boneless chicken breasts, thinly sliced
1 small red onion, thinly sliced
1 large clove garlic, pressed
¼ pound sliced portobello mushroom caps
2 tablespoons balsamic vinegar
1 8-ounce loaf ciabatta bread, cut crosswise into 4 pieces
¼ cup packed fresh basil leaves
1 cup shredded part-skim mozzarella cheese
½ cup diced avocado

1 Preheat broiler. Arrange sweet pepper halves on rack in broiler pan. Broil sweet pepper about 3 inches from the heat for 7 minutes or until skin blackens. Remove sweet pepper halves to bowl and cover with foil; set aside.

2 Meanwhile, in large skillet lightly sprayed with nonstick cooking spray cook chicken over medium-high heat for 6 minutes or until no longer pink, turning once. Remove chicken to platter; keep warm. Drain drippings from skillet and add onion and garlic; cook for 3 minutes. Add mushrooms; cook for 3 minutes or until tender, stirring occasionally. Stir in vinegar. Remove onion mixture to bowl; wipe out skillet.

3 Remove blackened skin from peppers. Cut into 1-inch strips. Add to bowl with onion mixture.

4 To assemble sandwiches: Cut each piece of bread in half horizontally. Divide onion mixture, chicken, and basil on bottom halves of bread. Place bread tops on each sandwich.

5 Heat skillet over medium heat. Place sandwiches in skillet. Weigh down with a smaller heavier skillet or foil-wrapped 1-pound cans. Or press sandwiches down with a large offset spatula. Cook sandwiches for 4 minutes or until bread is toasted, turning once. Remove bread top from each and divide cheese and avocado among sandwiches.

Makes 4 servings

COMPLETE MEAL SERVING
411 calories / 13 g total fat / 117 calories from fat / 29% calories from fat
65 mg cholesterol / 721 mg sodium / 43 g carbohydrate / 4 g fiber / 7 g sugars / 30 g protein

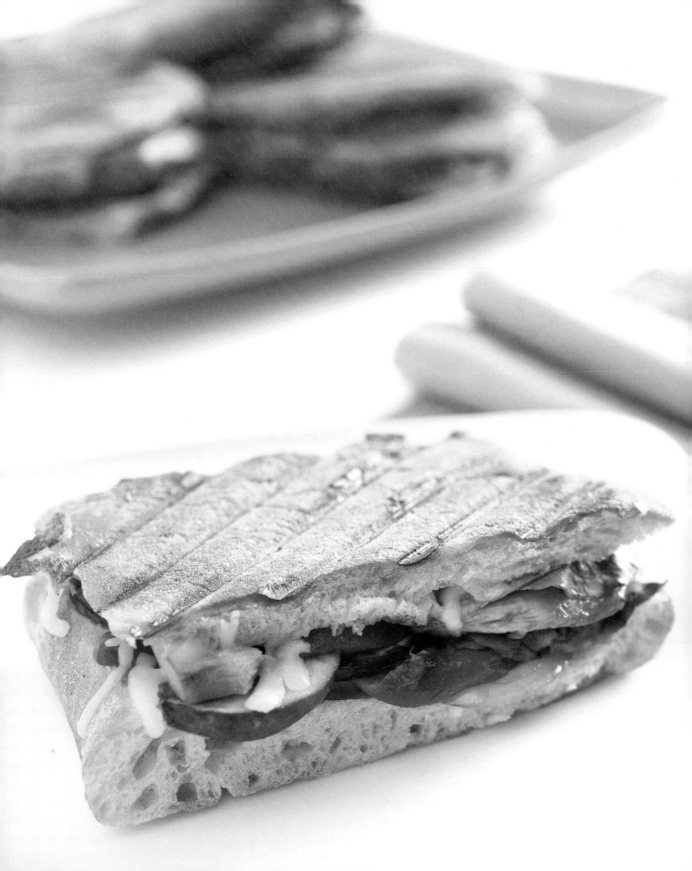

Grilled Chicken Burgers

Prep Time: 5 minutes ■ Cook Time: 10 minutes

Curry powder, green onion, and mint flavor these burgers with the tastes of the Middle East. A sweet yogurt sauce cools the spiciness.

1	pound ground chicken breast
1	Granny Smith apple, peeled, cored, grated, and squeezed dry with your hands
¼	cup chopped green onion (2)
2	tablespoons snipped fresh mint leaves
2	teaspoons curry powder
¼	teaspoon salt (optional)
¼	teaspoon cayenne pepper
	Nonstick cooking spray
1	cup low-fat plain yogurt
2	tablespoons mango chutney
4	romaine lettuce leaves, torn
4	6-inch whole wheat pitas, cut crosswise in half

1 In medium bowl combine chicken, apple, green onion, mint, curry powder, salt (if desired), and pepper. Shape into eight burgers.

2 Spray grill pan lightly with nonstick cooking spray. Heat over medium heat. Cook burgers for 10 minutes or until no longer pink, turning once.

3 Meanwhile, in bowl combine yogurt and chutney.

4 Divide lettuce among pitas. Place 1 burger in each pita half; divide yogurt sauce among pitas.

Makes 4 servings

COMPLETE MEAL SERVING
402 calories / 12 g total fat / 107 calories from fat / 27% calories from fat
78 mg cholesterol / 400 mg sodium / 51 g carbohydrate / 7 g fiber / 12 g sugars / 28 g protein

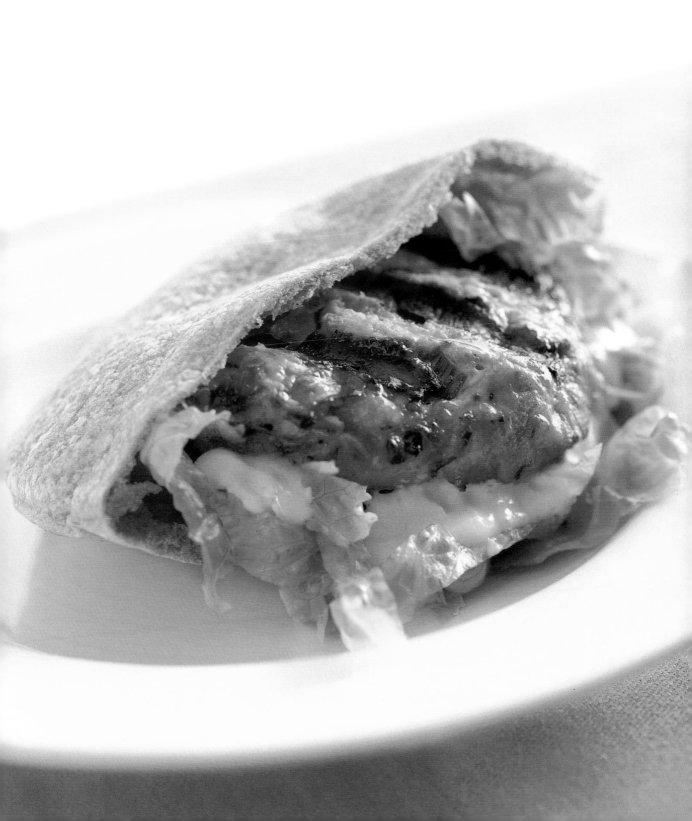

Barbecued Turkey Sandwiches

Prep Time: 10 minutes ■ Cook Time: 20 minutes

These sandwiches are a delicious way to use up cooked turkey, but cooked chicken will work just as well.

Nonstick cooking spray
2 medium yellow onions, thinly sliced
1 pound cooked turkey breast, shredded (4 cups)
½ cup barbecue sauce
⅓ cup tomato sauce
1 tablespoon chipotle peppers in adobo sauce, finely chopped (see tip, page 34)
½ 16-ounce bag shredded coleslaw mix (3 cups)
½ cup fat-free creamy coleslaw salad dressing
1¾ cups diced avocado
3 large whole wheat hoagie rolls, halved lengthwise, toasted

1 In medium skillet lightly sprayed with nonstick cooking spray cook onion over medium heat, stirring occasionally, for 15 minutes or until very tender. Add turkey, barbecue sauce, tomato sauce, and chipotle peppers in adobo sauce; bring to a simmer. Cook for 5 minutes to blend flavors.

2 Meanwhile, in medium bowl combine coleslaw mix and coleslaw dressing. Evenly divide turkey, coleslaw, and avocado among rolls.

Makes 6 servings

COMPLETE MEAL SERVING
411 calories / 13 g total fat / 114 calories from fat / 27% calories from fat
32 mg cholesterol / 1,463 mg sodium / 56 g carbohydrate / 10 g fiber / 10 g sugars / 22 g protein

Tuna and Veggie Pockets

Prep Time: 15 minutes

This recipe takes omega-3-rich canned tuna to a new level. Studded with red sweet pepper, shredded carrot, fennel, onion, and crunchy almonds, this tuna is bursting with nutritional benefits.

1	6-ounce can chunk light tuna in water, drained well
⅓	cup finely chopped red sweet pepper
⅓	cup shredded carrot
⅓	cup finely chopped fennel or celery
2	tablespoons chopped green onion (1)
3	tablespoons sliced almonds (approximately 1½ ounces)
1½	tablespoons reduced-fat mayonnaise
⅛	teaspoon ground black pepper
2	6-inch whole wheat pitas, halved crosswise
2	large romaine lettuce leaves, halved
1	small tomato, cut into 4 slices

1 In medium bowl combine tuna, sweet pepper, carrot, fennel, green onion, almonds, mayonnaise, and black pepper.

2 Open pita halves; place 1 lettuce half and 1 slice tomato in each. Divide tuna mixture among pita halves.

Makes 2 servings

COMPLETE MEAL SERVING
449 calories / 15 g total fat / 134 calories from fat / 28% calories from fat
26 mg cholesterol / 761 mg sodium / 48 g carbohydrate / 10 g fiber / 5 g sugars / 36 g protein

Roasted Vegetable Wraps

Prep Time: 20 minutes ■ Cook Time: 9 minutes

Baby bella mushrooms, also known as cremini, have a meaty, earthy flavor. They're about the same size as the white button mushrooms. Use them in recipes in which you'd prefer a rich mushroom presence.

	Nonstick cooking spray
2	cups zucchini, cut lengthwise in half, then sliced
1	cup sliced yellow sweet pepper
1	cup sliced baby bella mushrooms
⅔	cup red onion, cut into thin wedges
1	teaspoon ground cumin
1	teaspoon smoked paprika
¼	teaspoon grated lemon zest
4	8-inch whole wheat tortillas
2	teaspoons prepared hummus

1 Preheat oven to 450°F. Lightly spray jelly-roll pan with nonstick cooking spray.

2 Place zucchini, sweet pepper, mushrooms, onion, cumin, and paprika on pan. Roast for 8 minutes or until tender. Remove from oven; stir in zest.

3 Meanwhile, place tortillas on large microwave-safe plate. Cover with damp paper towel. Microwave on 100% power (high) 40 seconds or until tortillas are warm.

4 Place tortillas on work surface. Spread ½ teaspoon hummus in the center of each tortilla. Divide vegetables among tortillas. For each, fold top and bottom over. Fold one side up and over the filling, rolling until the filling is enclosed. Place 2 tortillas, seam sides down, on each of 2 plates.

Makes 2 servings

COMPLETE MEAL SERVING
447 calories / 15 g total fat / 138 calories from fat / 28% calories from fat
0 mg cholesterol / 1,037 mg sodium / 70 g carbohydrate / 13 g fiber / 8 g sugars / 18 g protein

Greek Pizza

Prep Time: 10 minutes ■ Cook Time: 18 minutes

The classic flavors of Greek cuisine—spinach, tomatoes, feta cheese, and olives—make a delicious variation to ordinary pizza. This one is sure to be a hit.

1   10-ounce prepared whole wheat pizza crust
    Nonstick cooking spray
1   cup chopped onion (1 large)
2   large cloves garlic, minced
1½ cups chopped red sweet pepper
1   9-ounce package baby spinach
1   tomato, cored and sliced
1   cup chopped kalamata olives
1   cup reduced-fat crumbled feta cheese

1 Preheat oven to 450°F. Place pizza crust on baking sheet.

2 In large nonstick skillet lightly sprayed with nonstick cooking spray cook onion, garlic, and sweet pepper over medium-high heat for 2 minutes, stirring occasionally. Add spinach and cook 8 minutes or until spinach wilts and liquid has evaporated.

3 Spread spinach mixture onto pizza crust. Arrange tomato and olives on spinach. Bake for 8 minutes or until heated through. Remove from oven and sprinkle with cheese. With a paper towel dab pizza to remove visible oil.

Makes 4 servings

COMPLETE MEAL SERVING
347 calories / 12 g total fat / 105 calories from fat / 29% calories from fat
25 mg cholesterol / 1,413 mg sodium / 49 g carbohydrate / 5 g fiber / 10 g sugars / 16 g protein

moving forward
Weight loss isn't a quick fix. Be patient and remember that long-term weight loss takes a long-term commitment.

Italian "Sausage" Pizza

Prep Time: 20 minutes ■ Cook Time: 17 minutes

When you're really working hard to cut calories but you're craving the flavors of spicy Italian sausage, try this quick mock version.

1	10-ounce prepared whole wheat thin pizza crust
¼	sweet onion, halved
1	clove garlic, halved
8	ounces skinless, boneless chicken breasts, cut into quarters
½	teaspoon fennel seeds, crushed
¼	teaspoon cracked black pepper
¼	teaspoon red pepper flakes
	Nonstick cooking spray
1	cup prepared pizza sauce
½	cup black olives, sliced
6	ounces shredded low-fat mozzarella cheese

1 Preheat oven to 450°F. Place pizza crust on baking sheet.

2 Place onion and garlic in food processor and pulse until minced. Add chicken, fennel seeds, black pepper, and red pepper flakes. Pulse until ground.

3 In large nonstick skillet lightly sprayed with nonstick cooking spray cook and stir chicken mixture over medium heat for 7 minutes or until brown and no longer pink.

4 Spread pizza sauce onto pizza crust. Top with chicken mixture. Bake for 10 minutes or until heated through. Remove from oven and sprinkle with olives and cheese. With a paper towel dab pizza to remove any visible oil.

Makes 4 servings

COMPLETE MEAL SERVING
439 calories / 12 g total fat / 109 calories from fat / 27% calories from fat
60 mg cholesterol / 1,147 mg sodium / 42 g carbohydrate / 3 g fiber / 6 g sugars / 31 g protein

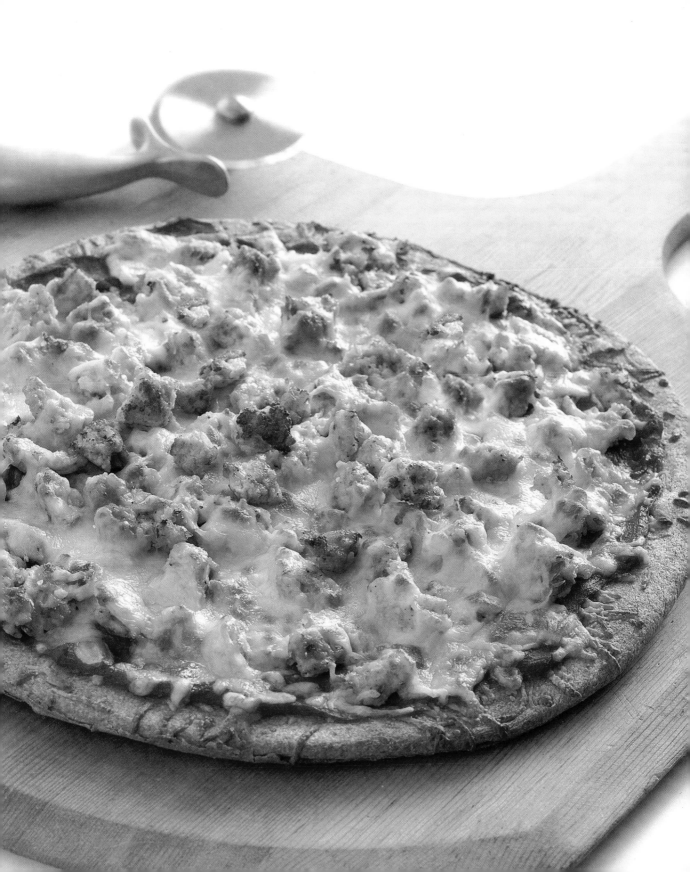

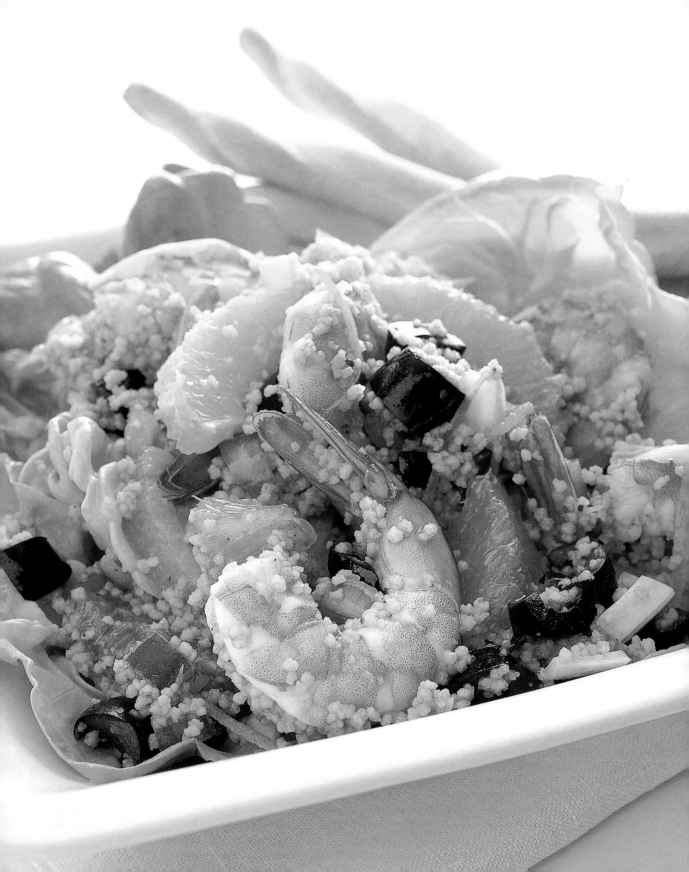

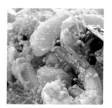

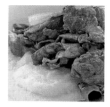

dinner

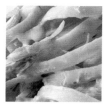

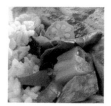

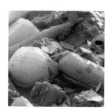

◄ *Citrus Shrimp and Couscous Toss, page 162*

POULTRY ENTRÉES

PORK ENTRÉES

BEEF, LAMB, AND VEAL ENTRÉES

FISH ENTRÉES

VEGETARIAN ENTRÉES

Thai Chicken Chowder

Prep Time: 10 minutes ■ Cook Time: 11 minutes

Step out of your comfort zone and try something deliciously new and exciting! Here mild coconut flavor mellows spicy soup for a rich, creamy taste. Look for curry paste in the ethnic section of your supermarket.

2   14½-ounce cans reduced-sodium chicken broth

2   cups reduced-fat (2%) milk

2   teaspoons coconut extract

2   tablespoons chopped fresh ginger

1   teaspoon red curry paste

1   1-pound bag frozen stir-fry vegetables without sauce

4   ounces straight-cut rice noodles

4   cups shredded cooked chicken breast (1 pound)

¼   cup snipped fresh cilantro

¼   cup lime juice

½   cup chopped unsalted dry-roasted peanuts

1 In large saucepan bring broth, milk, coconut extract, ginger, and curry paste to boiling over medium-high heat.

2 Add vegetables and rice noodles; cook for 10 minutes, stirring occasionally, until vegetables are crisp-tender and noodles are tender. Stir in chicken, cilantro, and lime juice; cook for 1 minute to heat through. Garnish with chopped peanuts.

Makes 4 servings

COMPLETE MEAL SERVING
516 calories / 15 g total fat / 135 calories from fat / 27% calories from fat
103 mg cholesterol / 771 mg sodium / 44 g carbohydrate / 5 g fiber / 10 g sugars / 49 g protein

moving forward
Log onto www.myalli.com for tips, support, and alli news.

Balsamic Roasted Chicken and Tomatoes

Prep Time: 10 minutes ■ Cook Time: 47 minutes

Sweet balsamic vinegar is the base of this rich, flavorful sauce. White balsamic vinegar keeps the color light, but if you have only the dark variety, use it and expect a slightly darker sauce.

	Nonstick cooking spray
½	cup white balsamic vinegar
3	tablespoons country-style Dijon mustard
3	tablespoons lemon juice
3	cloves garlic, chopped
3	tablespoons snipped fresh thyme
1	4-pound chicken, skinned and cut into eighths
6	plum tomatoes (1 pound), halved lengthwise
1	cup reduced-sodium chicken broth
½	cup pine nuts

1 Preheat oven to 400°F. Lightly spray large roasting pan with nonstick cooking spray.

2 Add vinegar, mustard, lemon juice, garlic, and thyme to prepared pan. Whisk to combine. Add chicken and toss to coat. Arrange chicken, flesh sides down, in balsamic mixture. Surround with tomato halves.

3 Roast for 40 minutes or until chicken is no longer pink (170°F for breasts, 180°F for thighs and drumsticks). Remove from oven. Raise oven rack to 3 inches from heat and increase oven temperature to broil. Turn chicken flesh sides up and broil for 2 minutes or until chicken is golden brown.

4 Place chicken and tomato halves on platter. Place roasting pan on burner over high heat. For gravy, whisk chicken broth into pan drippings, scraping up brown bits with wooden spoon. Cook, stirring, for 5 minutes or until reduced to ½ cup and slightly thickened. Serve gravy with chicken. Garnish with pine nuts.

Makes 6 servings

to complete the meal   For 6 servings: 12 ounces angel hair pasta, cooked ■ 6 cups romaine lettuce tossed with ⅓ cup fat-free Caesar salad dressing

COMPLETE MEAL SERVING
560 calories / 16 g total fat / 140 calories from fat / 25% calories from fat
103 mg cholesterol / 560 mg sodium / 57 g carbohydrate / 5 g fiber / 9 g sugars / 47 g protein

Barbecued Chicken with Stir-Fried Vegetables

Prep Time: 5 minutes ■ Cook Time: 25 minutes

This homemade barbecue sauce studded with vegetables is rich and flavorful. Served up with an order of stir-fried vegetables and brown rice, this meal is both satisfying and delicious.

	Nonstick cooking spray
¼	cup sliced celery
¼	cup thinly sliced green sweet pepper
¼	cup sliced onion
1	8-ounce can tomato sauce
¼	cup packed brown sugar
4	skinless, boneless chicken breast halves (1 pound)
¼	teaspoon ground black pepper
1	cup broccoli florets
1½	cups snow peas
1½	cups sliced carrot (3)
¾	cup shredded cheddar cheese
½	cup sliced black olives

1 Preheat oven to 350°F.

2 In small saucepan lightly sprayed with nonstick cooking spray cook and stir celery, sweet pepper, and onion over medium heat for 5 minutes or until tender. Add tomato sauce and sugar; bring to a simmer. Cover and simmer for 15 minutes.

3 Meanwhile, place chicken in roasting pan. Sprinkle with pepper. Bake for 15 minutes. Top with hot barbecue sauce and bake for 5 minutes longer or until no longer pink (170°F).

4 While chicken cooks, in large nonstick skillet lightly sprayed with nonstick cooking spray cook and stir broccoli, snow peas, and carrot over medium-high heat for 5 minutes or until vegetables are crisp-tender.

5 Remove chicken from oven; place on serving platter and divide cheese and olives over chicken. Serve with vegetables.

Makes 4 servings

to complete the meal   For 4 servings: 2 cups hot cooked quick-cooking brown rice

COMPLETE MEAL SERVING
392 calories / 12 g total fat / 108 calories from fat / 27% calories from fat
85 mg cholesterol / 725 mg sodium / 40 g carbohydrate / 5 g fiber / 22 g sugars / 33 g protein

Chicken and Artichoke Fricassee

Prep Time: 10 minutes ■ Cook Time: 30 minutes

A fricassee is a thick, hearty stew of chicken and vegetables that is often bathed in a heavy white sauce. Here's a healthier version, bursting with mushrooms, onion, and artichoke hearts in a rich tomato sauce flavored with olives.

3	tablespoons all-purpose flour
¼	teaspoon ground black pepper
1	pound skinless, boneless chicken thighs
	Nonstick cooking spray
1½	cups quartered baby bella mushrooms
1	cup chopped onion (1 large)
1	14½-ounce can diced tomatoes, undrained
1	14-ounce can artichoke hearts, drained and halved
¾	cup pitted kalamata olives

1 On sheet of waxed paper combine flour and pepper. Dredge chicken in flour mixture to coat, shaking off excess flour.

2 In large skillet lightly sprayed with nonstick cooking spray cook chicken over medium-high heat for 5 minutes, turning, until brown. Remove chicken to plate.

3 Add mushrooms and onion; cook for 5 minutes or until light brown. Add tomatoes, artichokes, and olives. Heat to boiling over high heat, stirring up any brown bits with spoon.

4 Return chicken to skillet. Reduce heat to medium-low; cover and simmer for 15 minutes or until chicken is no longer pink (170°F).

Makes 4 servings

to complete the meal For 4 servings: 6 ounces whole wheat noodles, cooked ■ one 1-pound package frozen broccoli, mushrooms, onions, and peppers, cooked

COMPLETE MEAL SERVING
501 calories / 15 g total fat / 135 calories from fat / 27% calories from fat
76 mg cholesterol / 963 mg sodium / 59 g carbohydrate / 9 g fiber / 11 g sugars / 33 g protein

Pollo en Mole Rojo

Prep Time: 5 minutes ■ Cook Time: 15 minutes

Mole literally means "concoction" and is a traditional dark red/brown Mexican sauce that's made from a blend of vegetables, spices, chiles, ground seeds, and sometimes chocolate. Look for red mole sauce in the ethnic section of your supermarket.

Nonstick cooking spray
2 pounds skinless, boneless chicken breasts, chopped
1 clove garlic, minced
4 tablespoons red mole sauce
1 cup fat-free, low-sodium chicken broth
1 cup prepared salsa
1 cup chopped avocado

1 In large skillet lightly sprayed with nonstick cooking spray cook and stir chicken, garlic, and mole sauce over medium heat for 5 minutes or until chicken is brown.

2 Add broth and bring to boiling. Reduce heat to low; cover and simmer for 10 minutes or until chicken is no longer pink. Stir in salsa. Top with avocado.

Makes 4 servings

to complete the meal For 4 servings: 2 cups hot cooked brown rice ■ 4 cups salad greens tossed with ½ cup fat-free ranch dressing

COMPLETE MEAL SERVING
515 calories / 14 g total fat / 127 calories from fat / 25% calories from fat
126 mg cholesterol / 909 mg sodium / 42 g carbohydrate / 6 g fiber / 5 g sugars / 51 g protein

moving forward
When shopping for groceries, stick to your shopping list to avoid impulse buying.

Chicken with Snap Peas

Prep Time: 5 minutes ■ Cook Time: 11 minutes

Adding whole grains to your diet is a great way to help with weight loss while adding essential nutrients. New whole grain products such as the noodles called for here are appearing on supermarket shelves daily. Try different brands and varieties of whole grain noodles, pastas, and breads to find ones that are right for your family.

6	ounces whole wheat blend wide egg noodles
1	pound sugar snap peas
1	red sweet pepper, cut into thin strips
⅔	cup orange juice
3	tablespoons hoisin sauce
3	tablespoons apple cider vinegar
2	tablespoons tomato sauce
1	pound skinless, boneless chicken breast, cut into 3-inch strips
3	tablespoons cornstarch
	Nonstick cooking spray
¾	cup dry-roasted unsalted cashews

1 Prepare noodles according to package directions, adding snap peas and sweet pepper 2 minutes before end of noodle cooking time. Drain.

2 Meanwhile, in small bowl stir together orange juice, hoisin sauce, vinegar, and tomato sauce.

3 In medium bowl toss chicken in cornstarch, shaking off excess cornstarch.

4 In large skillet lightly sprayed with nonstick cooking spray cook and stir half of the chicken over medium heat for 5 minutes or until light brown and no longer pink. With slotted spoon, remove chicken to bowl. Repeat with remaining chicken.

5 Return chicken and drippings to skillet; add orange juice mixture and bring to boiling. Add noodles, snap peas, and sweeet pepper; cook for 1 minute or until heated through. Place in serving bowl and sprinkle with cashews.

Makes 4 servings

COMPLETE MEAL SERVING
552 calories / 16 g total fat / 143 calories from fat / 26% calories from fat
63 mg cholesterol / 321 mg sodium / 66 g carbohydrate / 9 g fiber / 14 g sugars / 36 g protein

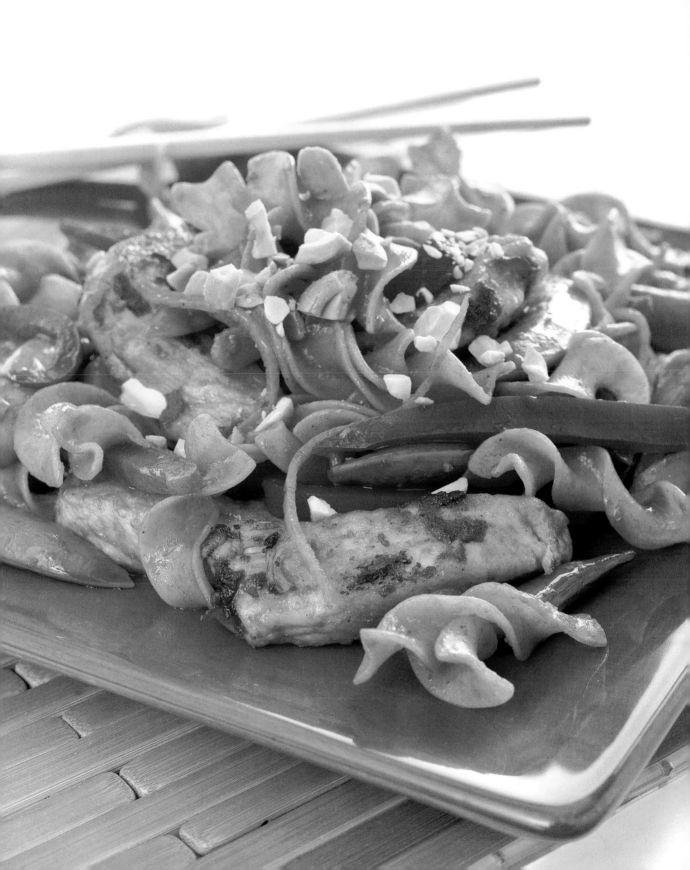

Chicken with Tomatoes, Olives, and Feta

Prep Time: 5 minutes ■ Cook Time: 24 minutes

For a quick and easy way to seed a tomato, cut the tomato in half crosswise. With your finger or a small spoon, scoop the seeds out and discard.

4	skinless, boneless chicken breast halves (1 pound)
1	teaspoon Greek seasoning blend, crushed
	Nonstick cooking spray
1	red onion, cut into ¼-inch slices
1	clove garlic, minced
3	medium tomatoes, seeded and chopped
1	cup low-sodium chicken broth
½	cup kalamata olives
4	ounces reduced-fat feta cheese, crumbled

1 Season chicken with seasoning blend.

2 In large nonstick skillet lightly sprayed with nonstick cooking spray cook chicken over medium heat for 5 minutes or until brown, turning once. Remove to plate; keep warm.

3 Add onion; cook and stir for 3 minutes. Add garlic and tomato; cook and stir for 5 minutes. Add broth and bring to simmer. Return chicken to skillet, cover, and simmer for 8 minutes or until chicken is no longer pink (170°F).

4 Place chicken on plate. Increase heat to high and boil broth mixture for 3 minutes or until thickened. Stir in olives. Spoon sauce over chicken and sprinkle with cheese.

Makes 4 servings

to complete the meal For 4 servings: 2 cups hot cooked orzo tossed with 1 tablespoon snipped fresh parsley ■ 6 cups baby arugula tossed with ½ cup fat-free red wine vinaigrette and topped with 2 tablespoons pine nuts

COMPLETE MEAL SERVING
391 calories / 12 g total fat / 110 calories from fat / 28% calories from fat
74 mg cholesterol / 985 mg sodium / 36 g carbohydrate / 3 g fiber / 9 g sugars / 36 g protein

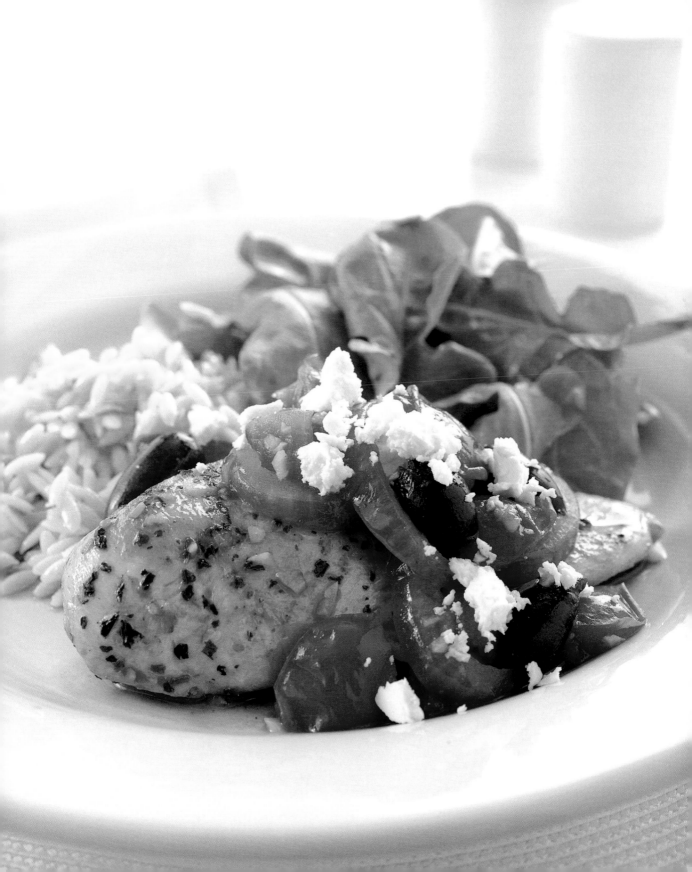

Chicken in Red Wine Sauce

Prep Time: 5 minutes ■ Cook Time: 23 minutes

When purchasing wine for cooking, always go for a wine you'd enjoy drinking. Avoid "cooking wine" sold in the condiment section of your supermarket because it contains sodium and is inferior in flavor.

2	tablespoons all-purpose flour
½	teaspoon ground black pepper
¼	teaspoon salt
1	pound thinly sliced chicken cutlets
	Nonstick cooking spray
1	10-ounce package sliced white mushrooms
1	teaspoon olive oil
1	cup Merlot, Gamay, or Pinot Noir wine
1	cup cranberry juice

1 In large resealable plastic bag combine flour, pepper, and salt. Dredge chicken in flour mixture, shaking off excess.

2 In large nonstick skillet lightly sprayed with nonstick cooking spray cook half the chicken over medium-high heat for 5 minutes or until light brown; remove to plate. Repeat with remaining chicken.

3 In same skillet cook mushrooms in hot oil for 5 minutes or until mushrooms are golden brown, stirring occasionally; remove to plate with chicken.

4 Add wine and cranberry juice and stir to scrape up any browned bits. Bring to boiling over high heat. Cook for 5 minutes or until reduced to 1 cup. Cook and stir over medium-high heat for 3 minutes until sauce thickens. Add chicken and mushrooms and cook for 1 minute or until heated through.

Makes 4 servings

to complete the meal   For 4 servings: 4 medium potatoes, baked, with 4 tablespoons low-fat sour cream ■ 6 cups mesclun tossed with ⅓ cup fat-free Italian dressing, ½ cup shredded reduced-fat Swiss cheese, and ¼ cup slivered almonds

COMPLETE MEAL SERVING
511 calories / 15 g total fat / 131 calories from fat / 25% calories from fat
79 mg cholesterol / 568 mg sodium / 60 g carbohydrate / 8 g fiber / 14 g sugars / 37 g protein

Taquitos Suaves Sonorenses

Prep Time: 5 minutes ■ Cook Time: 16 minutes

This Mexican-inspired dish is bursting with flavor. For a zestier version, opt for low-fat pepper Jack cheese in place of the Monterey Jack.

1	pound cooked chicken breast, chopped
4	cups torn romaine lettuce
1½	cups mild salsa
1	cup shredded low-fat Monterey Jack cheese
2	tablespoons snipped fresh cilantro
1	medium avocado, halved, pitted, peeled, and chopped
8	6-inch corn tortillas

1 In large bowl combine chicken, lettuce, salsa, cheese, cilantro, and avocado. Gently toss to coat.

2 Heat large nonstick skillet over medium heat. Add tortillas, 1 at a time, and cook for 2 minutes or until hot, turning once.

3 Place 2 tortillas on each of 4 plates. Divide chicken mixture among the tortillas and fold in half.

Makes 4 servings

COMPLETE MEAL SERVING
403 calories / 12 g total fat / 111 calories from fat / 27% calories from fat
73 mg cholesterol / 976 mg sodium / 40 g carbohydrate / 7 g fiber / 7 g sugars / 37 g protein

moving forward

Saying "no" to tempting foods might seem hard, but it's harder to keep battling the weight.

Chicken Potocino

Prep Time: 8 minutes ■ Cook Time: 11 minutes

Green salsa, also known as salsa verde, contains tomatillos, a Mexican relative of the tomato that looks like small green tomatoes covered with parchment-like husks. Find tomatillos in the produce section of the supermarket. Look for green salsa in the ethnic section or along with the salsas.

Nonstick cooking spray
1 pound skinless, boneless chicken breasts, cut into ¼-inch strips
1 small onion, sliced
1 jalapeño pepper, seeded and sliced (see tip, page 34)
2 leaves snipped fresh basil
1 clove garlic, minced
1 teaspoon dried oregano, crushed
1 cup mild green salsa
½ cup crushed tomatoes
½ cup diced avocado

1 In medium skillet lightly sprayed with nonstick cooking spray cook chicken and onion over medium heat for 5 minutes or until light brown.

2 Add jalapeño, basil, garlic, and oregano; cook for 1 minute. Add salsa and tomatoes; cook and stir for 5 minutes or until chicken is no longer pink. Garnish with avocado.

Makes 4 servings

to complete the meal For 4 servings: 2 cups hot cooked quick-cooking brown rice ■ 1 pound frozen green beans, steamed and topped with ½ cup toasted almonds

COMPLETE MEAL SERVING
415 calories / 13 g total fat / 119 calories from fat / 28% calories from fat
63 mg cholesterol / 435 mg sodium / 44 g carbohydrate / 8 g fiber / 5 g sugars / 32 g protein

Slow Cooker Chicken Cacciatore

Prep Time: 10 minutes ■ Cook Time: 3 to 4 hours (high), 6 to 8 hours (low)

This hearty classic chicken recipe features chicken thighs cooked with onions and green and red sweet peppers in a rich tomato sauce. Turn it on first thing in the morning and you'll have dinner ready when you are.

1	cup chopped onion (1 large)
3	cloves garlic, minced
2	tablespoons all-purpose flour
¼	teaspoon crushed red pepper flakes
1	cup chopped red sweet pepper (1 large)
1	cup chopped green sweet pepper (1 large)
2	pounds skinless, boneless chicken thighs, trimmed of any visible fat
1	26-ounce jar low-sodium marinara sauce
½	cup shredded fat-free Parmesan cheese

1 Place onion, garlic, flour, and pepper flakes in a 3½- to 4-quart slow cooker. Stir until flour coats the onion.

2 Layer sweet peppers, chicken, and marinara sauce on top. Cover and cook on low-heat setting for 6 to 8 hours or on high-heat setting for 3 to 4 hours until chicken and vegetables are fork-tender.

3 Stir well and place in serving bowl. Sprinkle with cheese.

Makes 6 servings

to complete the meal Per serving: one 1½-ounce whole wheat roll

COMPLETE MEAL SERVING
428 calories / 14 g total fat / 127 calories from fat / 30% calories from fat
101 mg cholesterol / 518 mg sodium / 37 g carbohydrate / 6 g fiber / 10 g sugars / 36 g protein

Honey Mustard Baked Chicken Wings

Prep Time: 10 minutes ■ Cook Time: 30 minutes

You don't have to be a fan of football to enjoy tailgate food, and you don't have to feel linebacker-size guilt for indulging in it either. Slimmed down and simplified, these chicken wings are the real deal.

6	tablespoons honey Dijon mustard
2	tablespoons lemon juice
½	teaspoon ground black pepper
16	chicken drummettes, skinned

1 Preheat oven to 400°F. Line jelly-roll pan with foil. Place rack in pan.

2 In large bowl combine mustard, lemon juice, and pepper. Add drummettes; toss to coat well.

3 Place on rack in pan. Roast for 30 minutes, turning once, until chicken is no longer pink.

Makes 4 servings

to complete the meal   For 4 servings: 12 ounces baked crinkle-cut frozen french fries
■ one 16-ounce package coleslaw tossed with
½ cup fat-free mayonnaise

COMPLETE MEAL SERVING
423 calories / 14 g total fat / 126 calories from fat / 30% calories from fat
71 mg cholesterol / 431 mg sodium / 43 g carbohydrate / 5 g fiber / 19 g sugars / 29 g protein

moving forward
On the weekends, stay on track by planning a social
calendar that doesn't revolve around food.

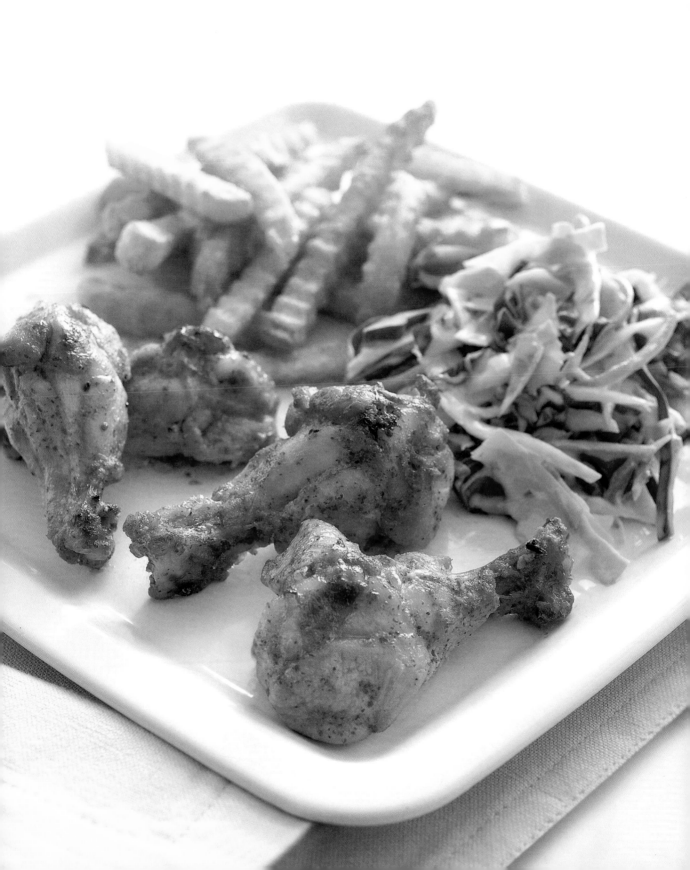

Lemon Roasted Chicken

Prep Time: 10 minutes ■ Cook Time: 1½ hours

For a perfect Sunday dinner, roast chicken, baked potatoes, and steamed vegetables are sure winners. Be sure to remove the skin from the chicken because it's loaded with fat and not included in the nutrition analyses throughout this book.

¼ cup assorted snipped fresh herbs, such as parsley, thyme, marjoram, and rosemary
2 cloves garlic, minced
¼ teaspoon ground black pepper
1 lemon
1 4-pound whole broiler chicken

1 Preheat oven to 350°F.

2 In small bowl combine herbs, garlic, and pepper.

3 Cut 4 thin slices from half of lemon, remove any seeds, and cut each slice in half. Set aside. From remaining lemon half, squeeze 1 tablespoon juice and stir into herb mixture.

4 Place chicken, breast side up, on rack in roasting pan. Using hands, gently loosen skin from breast on both sides, forming 2 pockets. Slide lemon slices and herb mixture under skin.

5 Roast chicken for 1½ hours or until drumsticks move easily in their sockets and chicken is no longer pink (180°F). Remove chicken from oven. Cover; let stand for 10 minutes before slicing. Remove and discard skin before serving.

Makes 6 servings

to complete the meal For 6 servings: 6 medium potatoes, baked, with 6 tablespoons low-fat sour cream ■ one 16-ounce package broccoli, cauliflower, and peppers, cooked and sprinkled with 6 tablespoons shredded low-fat cheddar cheese

COMPLETE MEAL SERVING
445 calories / 12 g total fat / 108 calories from fat / 25% calories from fat
110 mg cholesterol / 158 mg sodium / 43 g carbohydrate / 6 g fiber / 4 g sugars / 40 g protein

Spicy Chicken in Lettuce Cups

Prep Time: 10 minutes ■ Cook Time: 5 minutes

When purchasing ground chicken, opting for ground chicken breast, sometimes called ground white meat chicken, will give you the lowest fat content. Otherwise you may end up with ground dark meat and skin, yielding a much higher fat content.

1½	pounds ground chicken breast
1	cup chopped red sweet pepper (1 large)
¼	cup chopped green onion (2)
2	tablespoons reduced-sodium soy sauce
2	tablespoons seasoned rice wine vinegar
1	clove garlic, minced
1	tablespoon chopped fresh ginger
¼	teaspoon crushed red pepper flakes
	Nonstick cooking spray
2	cups cooked brown rice
½	cup chopped unsalted dry-roasted peanuts
2	tablespoons snipped fresh cilantro
12	Boston lettuce leaves

1 In large bowl combine chicken, sweet pepper, green onion, soy sauce, vinegar, garlic, ginger, and pepper flakes.

2 In large nonstick skillet lightly sprayed with nonstick cooking spray cook and stir chicken mixture over medium-high heat for 5 minutes or until chicken is no longer pink. Stir in rice, peanuts, and cilantro. Place 3 lettuce leaves onto each of 4 plates. Divide chicken mixture among lettuce leaves. Roll up to eat.

Makes 4 servings

COMPLETE MEAL SERVING
428 calories / 14 g total fat / 127 calories from fat / 30% calories from fat
94 mg cholesterol / 542 mg sodium / 33 g carbohydrate / 5 g fiber / 4 g sugars / 43 g protein

Polenta, Chicken, and Swiss Chard

Prep Time: 10 minutes ■ Cook Time: 10 minutes

Polenta is a cornmeal mush that is common in northern Italian cooking. Traditionally it cooks on the stovetop with constant stirring for 40 minutes. Here instant polenta cuts that time down to 3 minutes, making this a comfort-food meal ready in just 20 minutes.

1 cup instant polenta
4 ounces goat cheese (chèvre)
  Nonstick cooking spray
1 pound skinless, boneless chicken breasts, cut into thin strips
4 cups very loosely packed roughly chopped Swiss chard or baby spinach leaves

1 In medium saucepan prepare the polenta according to package directions. Stir in cheese. Pour into large serving bowl.

2 Meanwhile, in nonstick skillet lightly sprayed with nonstick cooking spray cook and stir chicken over medium heat for 5 minutes or until brown. Add Swiss chard and cook, stirring, about 5 minutes or until chard is tender and chicken is no longer pink. Place over the polenta.

Makes 4 servings

to complete the meal   For 4 servings: 4 cups torn green lettuce tossed with 1 green apple, cored and cut into thin strips, and drizzled with ⅓ cup fat-free balsamic vinaigrette, topped with ¼ cup pecan halves

COMPLETE MEAL SERVING
487 calories / 16 g total fat / 146 calories from fat / 30% calories from fat
85 mg cholesterol / 438 mg sodium / 51 g carbohydrate / 8 g fiber / 8 g sugars / 35 g protein

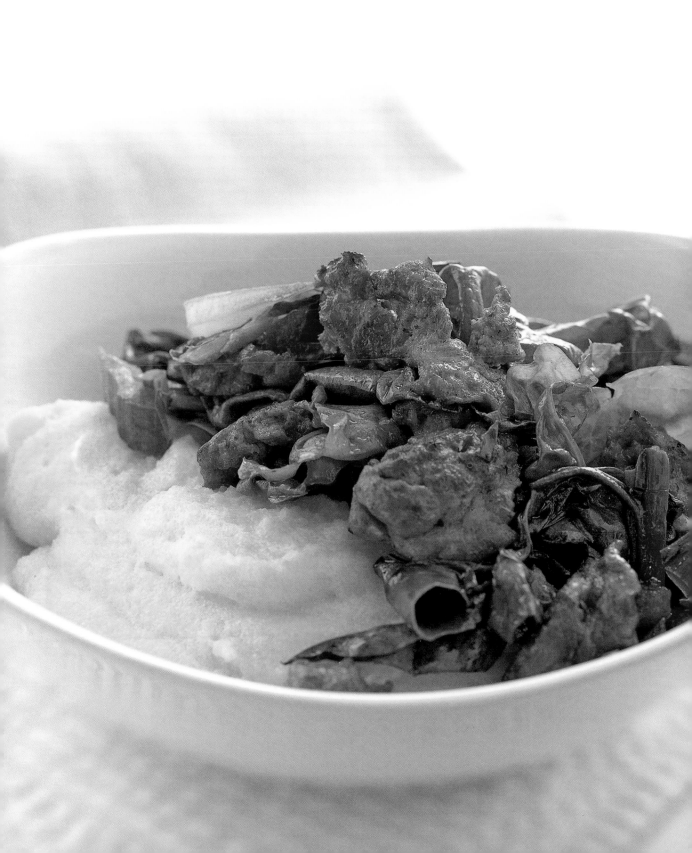

Thai Chicken Patties

Prep Time: 20 minutes ■ Cook Time: 8 minutes

These savory chicken patties are perfect for easy entertaining. Make them in advance through step 1, refrigerate, then lightly brown patties while you mingle in the kitchen with guests.

1½	pounds ground chicken breast
⅓	cup panko (Japanese bread crumbs)
½	cup chopped red and/or yellow sweet pepper
1	egg white
1	tablespoon chopped fresh ginger
1	tablespoon snipped fresh cilantro
1	clove garlic, minced
1	teaspoon packed brown sugar
¼	teaspoon ground black pepper
½	cup chopped peanuts

1 In large bowl mix together chicken, panko, sweet pepper, egg white, ginger, cilantro, garlic, brown sugar, and black pepper. Shape into 4 patties.

2 In large nonstick skillet lightly sprayed with nonstick cooking spray cook patties over medium-high heat for 8 minutes or until brown and no longer pink, turning once. Garnish with peanuts.

Makes 4 servings

to complete the meal For 4 servings: 4 cups torn red leaf lettuce tossed with 1 orange sweet pepper, cut into thin strips; 1 cucumber, peeled, seeded, and cut into thin strips; and ⅓ cup creamy fat-free French salad dressing ■ 2 cups hot cooked brown rice

COMPLETE MEAL SERVING
474 calories / 14 g total fat / 125 calories from fat / 26% calories from fat
94 mg cholesterol / 355 mg sodium / 46 g carbohydrate / 7 g fiber / 9 g sugars / 42 g protein

Turkey-Vegetable Saute

Prep Time: 10 minutes ■ Cook Time: 11 minutes

Crush dried herbs before adding them to a dish to release their flavor. Simply rub them between your hands before adding them to the pan.

Nonstick cooking spray

1	cup chopped onion (1 medium)
1½	pounds turkey breast strips
8	ounces asparagus, cut into 1½-inch pieces
6	ounces sliced baby bella or white mushrooms
½	teaspoon dried sage, crushed
½	teaspoon dried rosemary, crushed
1	teaspoon salt
⅛	teaspoon ground black pepper
¼	cup low-sodium chicken broth
¼	cup sour cream
¼	cup sliced almonds

1 In large skillet lightly sprayed with nonstick cooking spray cook onion over medium heat for 5 minutes or until tender, stirring occasionally.

2 Add turkey and cook for 1 minute or until golden. Add asparagus, mushrooms, sage, rosemary, salt, and pepper. Cook, stirring, for 3 minutes.

3 Add broth; cover and simmer for 2 minutes or until asparagus is crisp-tender and turkey is no longer pink. Remove from heat and stir in sour cream. Garnish with almonds.

Makes 4 servings

to complete the meal For 4 servings: 2 cups hot cooked whole wheat noodles tossed with ½ cup shredded cheddar cheese

COMPLETE MEAL SERVING
381 calories / 12 g total fat / 111 calories from fat / 28% calories from fat
96 mg cholesterol / 159 mg sodium / 30 g carbohydrate / 6 g fiber / 5 g sugars / 40 g protein

Turkey Scaloppine Provençal

Prep Time: 10 minutes ■ Cook Time: 15 minutes

Tomatoes, olives, and garlic combine to make a classic Provençal sauce, which is delicious on top of tender turkey cutlets. Strong, bold flavors like these make meals satisfying and delightful.

- 4 turkey breast cutlets (1 pound)
- 3 tablespoons all-purpose flour
- ⅛ teaspoon ground black pepper
  Nonstick cooking spray
- 1 14½-ounce can diced tomatoes with garlic and onion, undrained
- 1 cup pitted ripe or green olives, sliced
- ¼ cup dry white wine
- ½ cup pine nuts

1 Place turkey between two sheets of waxed paper on hard surface. Pound gently with bottom of heavy saucepan or skillet or flat side of meat mallet to flatten slightly.

2 In large resealable plastic bag combine flour and pepper. Add turkey; seal and toss to coat.

3 In large skillet lightly sprayed with nonstick cooking spray cook turkey over medium heat for 5 minutes or until golden, turning once. Place on serving plate and keep warm.

4 Add tomatoes, olives, and wine to the skillet. Bring to a simmer over medium-high heat. Reduce heat to medium-low and simmer for 10 minutes. Serve the sauce over turkey. Garnish with pine nuts.

Makes 4 servings

to complete the meal For 4 servings: 2 cups hot cooked orzo pasta, ⅓ cup grated Parmesan cheese
■ 1 pound green beans, steamed

COMPLETE MEAL SERVING
413 calories / 12 g total fat / 109 calories from fat / 26% calories from fat
80 mg cholesterol / 965 mg sodium / 40 g carbohydrate / 7 g fiber / 9 g sugars / 39 g protein

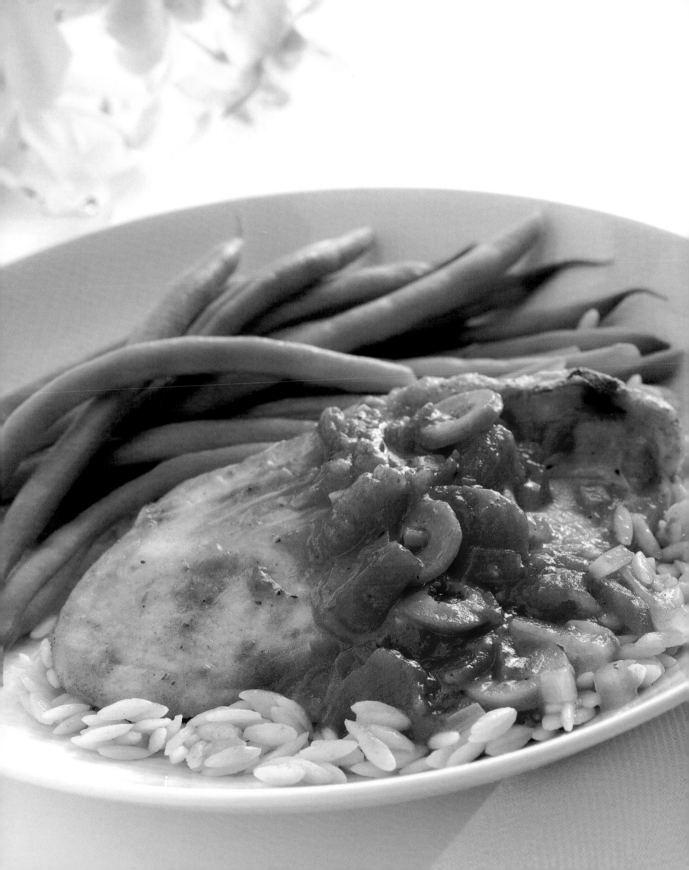

Sweet Potato Hash with Turkey

Prep Time: 15 minutes ■ Cook Time: 20 minutes

When selecting ground turkey, be sure to reach for ground turkey breast (or white meat). Otherwise you may end up with ground meat that contains dark meat as well as some skin, both adding extra fat.

1½	pounds sweet potatoes, peeled and chopped (about 5 cups)
2	cups water
	Nonstick cooking spray
1	cup chopped red onion (1 medium)
1	pound ground turkey breast
½	cup orange juice
½	teaspoon ground cinnamon
½	teaspoon ground cumin
⅓	cup chopped walnuts

1 In medium microwave-safe bowl combine sweet potato and the water. Cover and microwave on 100% power (high) for 10 minutes or until potato is tender. Drain potato; set aside.

2 Meanwhile, in large nonstick skillet lightly sprayed with nonstick cooking spray cook and stir onion over medium-high heat for 3 minutes. Add ground turkey and cook, stirring occasionally to crumble, 7 minutes or until turkey is no longer pink. Add cooked potatoes, orange juice, cinnamon, and cumin. Cook, stirring, for 10 minutes or until potatoes are brown. Garnish with chopped walnuts.

Makes 4 servings

to complete the meal   For 4 servings: 6 cups salad greens tossed with ½ cup shredded cheddar cheese and ⅓ cup fat-free Italian vinaigrette

COMPLETE MEAL SERVING
453 calories / 13 g total fat / 113 calories from fat / 25% calories from fat
89 mg cholesterol / 373 mg sodium / 50 g carbohydrate / 6 g fiber / 26 g sugars / 36 g protein

moving forward
Dance the weight away. Get moving to your favorite music anytime.

Tex-Mex Mini Meat Loaves

Prep Time: 5 minutes ■ Cook Time: 20 minutes

Cooking meat loaves in muffin cups helps get dinner on the table fast. These flavorful bites are fun for kids of all ages.

	Nonstick cooking spray
1	pound ground turkey breast
¾	cup rolled oats
½	cup mild red salsa
¼	cup snipped fresh cilantro
2	egg whites
2	teaspoons chili powder
1½	teaspoons ground cumin
¾	cup mild chunky salsa
½	cup low-fat cheddar cheese

1 Preheat oven to 400°F. Lightly spray 12-cup muffin pan with nonstick cooking spray.

2 In large bowl combine turkey, oats, red salsa, cilantro, egg whites, chili powder, and cumin. Divide mixture among muffin cups.

3 Bake for 20 minutes or until no longer pink (165°F).

4 Place 2 mini meat loaves on each of 6 plates. Top each meat loaf with 1 tablespoon chunky salsa and 2 teaspoons cheese.

Makes 6 servings

to complete the meal For 6 servings: 3 cups hot cooked instant brown rice tossed with 6 tablespoons chopped pecans ■ 1½ pounds green beans, steamed

COMPLETE MEAL SERVING
376 calories / 12 g total fat / 107 calories from fat / 28% calories from fat
35 mg cholesterol / 514 mg sodium / 47 g carbohydrate / 7 g fiber / 4 g sugars / 22 g protein

Turkey and Sweet Potato Stew

Prep Time: 5 minutes ■ Cook Time: 25 minutes

Sweet potatoes are a great addition to healthy meal plans. A good source of fiber and vitamin C, they're bursting with beta-carotene. Opt for the darkest ones because they contain the most vitamins.

Nonstick cooking spray
1   medium sweet potato (12 ounces), cut into ½-inch cubes
1   cup chopped onion (1 large)
1   28-ounce can no-salt-added whole peeled tomatoes in thick puree, coarsely chopped
3   cups shredded cooked turkey breast (12 ounces)
1   tablespoon chipotle pepper in adobo sauce
1   teaspoon dried oregano, crushed
2   teaspoons packed brown sugar
2   tablespoons snipped fresh cilantro
1   cup diced avocado
¼   cup sour cream

1 In Dutch oven lightly sprayed with nonstick cooking spray cook and stir sweet potato and onion over medium-high heat for 5 minutes or until light brown.

2 Reduce heat to medium and add tomatoes, turkey, chipotle pepper, oregano, and brown sugar. Bring to boiling, stirring frequently.

3 Reduce heat to low; cover and simmer for 20 minutes to blend flavors. Stir in cilantro and avocado. Divide stew among 4 bowls and dollop 1 tablespoon of sour cream over each serving.

Makes 4 servings

to complete the meal   For 4 servings: 6 cups salad greens tossed with ½ cup fat-free Italian dressing, topped with ¼ cup shredded reduced-fat cheddar cheese

COMPLETE MEAL SERVING
384 calories / 12 g total fat / 107 calories from fat / 27% calories from fat
83 mg cholesterol / 648 mg sodium / 38 g carbohydrate / 8 g fiber / 20 g sugars / 33 g protein

Roasted Pork Tenderloin with Autumn Vegetables

Prep Time: 10 minutes ■ Cook Time: 20 minutes

Tender, juicy pork tenderloin comes to life when brushed with mustard and sprinkled with herbes de Provence. This herb blend usually includes basil, fennel seeds, lavender, rosemary, sage, thyme, and marjoram. Look for it in small crocks or tins. A great alternative is a French herb roasting rub, which you'll find in the spice section of your grocery store.

	Nonstick cooking spray
1	butternut squash (1½ pounds), peeled, halved, seeded, and cut into 1-inch pieces
2	sweet potatoes (18 ounces), peeled and cut into ½-inch slices
1	Granny Smith apple, peeled, cored, and cut into 6 pieces
1	parsnip, peeled and bias-sliced
1	large red onion, cut into ½-inch wedges
1	green sweet pepper, cut into ½-inch pieces
1	teaspoon olive oil
½	teaspoon ground black pepper
2	1-pound pork tenderloins
2	tablespoons Dijon mustard
1	tablespoon herbes de Provence, crushed
6	tablespoons chopped pecans

1 Preheat oven to 500°F. Lightly spray jelly-roll pan with nonstick cooking spray.

2 In large bowl combine squash, sweet potato, apple, parsnip, onion, sweet pepper, oil, and black pepper.

3 Arrange vegetables in single layer in prepared pan.

4 Lightly spray small roasting pan with nonstick cooking spray. Place pork in roasting pan. Brush with mustard and sprinkle with herbes de Provence. Place both pans in oven and roast for 20 minutes or until vegetables are tender and meat thermometer registers 155°F in pork. Sprinkle chopped pecans over vegetables.

Makes 6 servings

to complete the meal   Per serving: one 1-ounce whole wheat dinner roll with
1 teaspoon trans-fat-free canola margarine

COMPLETE MEAL SERVING
450 calories / 15 g total fat / 134 calories from fat / 29% calories from fat
86 mg cholesterol / 332 mg sodium / 46 g carbohydrate / 9 g fiber / 14 g sugars / 36 g protein

Blackberry Pork Tenderloin

Prep Time: 15 minutes ▪ Cook Time: 10 minutes

Mild, juicy pork tenderloin is a lean cut of meat—as lean as a chicken breast. Think "loin" equals "lean" when selecting cuts. Pork tenderloin, as the name suggests, is very tender and works well when grilled, broiled, or sauteed.

4	cloves garlic, minced
1	teaspoon ground black pepper
1	1-pound pork tenderloin
1	cup white wine
1	cup water
2	tablespoons lime juice
¼	cup packed brown sugar
1	pound fresh blackberries

1 Preheat broiler.

2 In small bowl combine garlic and pepper. Place tenderloin on rack in broiler pan. Rub garlic mixture over tenderloin. Let stand for 10 minutes.

3 Broil pork 5 inches from heat for 10 minutes or until meat thermometer registers 155°F. Let stand for 5 minutes before slicing.

4 Meanwhile, in medium saucepan boil wine, the water, lime juice, brown sugar, and blackberries for 5 minutes or until slightly thickened. Serve with pork.

Makes 4 servings

to complete the meal For 4 servings: 8 ounces hot cooked whole grain angel hair pasta tossed with ½ cup grated Parmesan and 1 tablespoon snipped fresh parsley ▪ 1 pound asparagus, steamed and topped with 2 teaspoons trans-fat-free canola margarine

COMPLETE MEAL SERVING
435 calories / 13 g total fat / 113 calories from fat / 25% calories from fat
85 mg cholesterol / 270 mg sodium / 48 g carbohydrate / 10 g fiber / 24 g sugars / 35 g protein

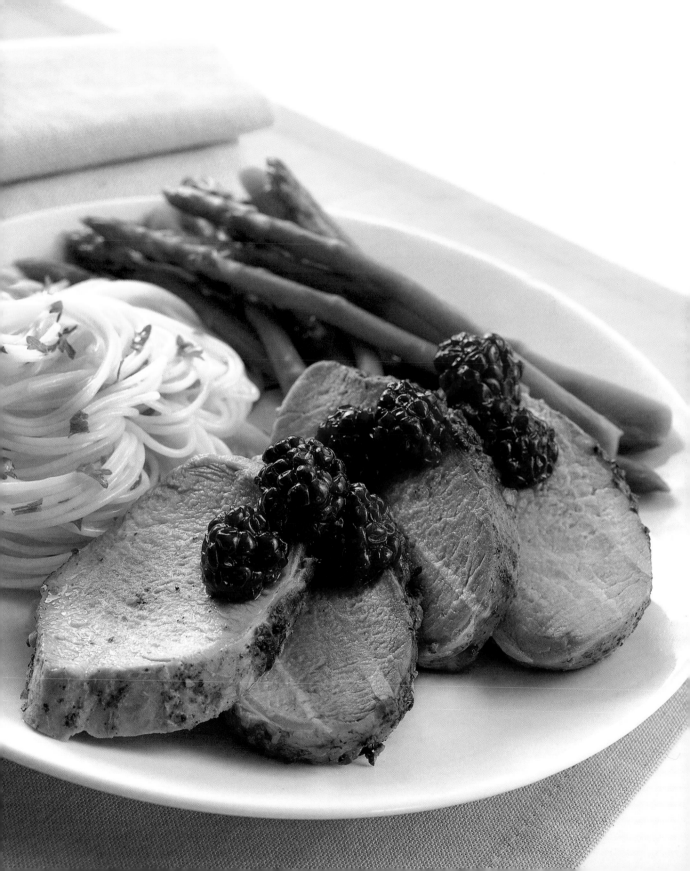

Rosemary Pork Roast

Prep Time: 5 minutes ■ Cook Time: 1 hour

This meal is just right for a weekend dinner. The prep time you'll spend in the kitchen is minimal, and the roast cooks on its own. Relax while it fills your home with an appetizing aroma.

1 2½-pound boneless pork loin roast, trimmed
2 cloves garlic, minced
1 tablespoon balsamic vinegar
1 tablespoon snipped fresh rosemary leaves
¼ teaspoon salt
⅛ teaspoon ground black pepper

1 Preheat oven to 400°F.

2 Place roast on rack in shallow roasting pan.

3 In small bowl combine garlic, vinegar, rosemary, salt, and pepper. Rub mixture over pork.

4 Roast for 1 hour or until meat thermometer registers 150°F. Let stand 10 minutes before slicing. The temperature of the meat after standing should be 160°F.

Makes 8 servings

to complete the meal Per serving: 1 baked sweet potato topped with 1 tablespoon sour cream
■ ½ cup applesauce

COMPLETE MEAL SERVING
402 calories / 12 g total fat / 110 calories from fat / 27% calories from fat
85 mg cholesterol / 161 mg sodium / 43 g carbohydrate / 5 g fiber / 24 g sugars / 30 g protein

moving forward
Don't go it alone. Connect with other alli users on the alli message board on www.myalli.com.

Pork and Pepper Stir-Fry

Prep Time: 5 minutes ▪ Cook Time: 12 minutes

This zesty meal comes together in minutes for a delicious, healthful option that's faster than takeout. Served over quick-cooking rice, it's sure to become a family favorite.

- ¼ cup orange juice
- ¼ cup prepared stir-fry sauce
  Nonstick cooking spray
- 1 1-pound pork tenderloin, trimmed and cut into thin strips
- ½ 1-pound bag frozen mixed pepper stir-fry
- 8 ounces bean sprouts
- 2 tablespoons sesame seeds, toasted

1 In small bowl stir together orange juice and stir-fry sauce.

2 In large nonstick skillet lightly sprayed with nonstick cooking spray cook and stir pork over medium-high heat for 5 minutes or until no pink remains. Remove to bowl.

3 Add frozen pepper stir-fry and sprouts to skillet; cook and stir for 5 minutes or until crisp-tender. Return pork to skillet and stir in orange juice mixture; heat through. Sprinkle with sesame seeds.

Makes 4 servings

to complete the meal For 4 servings: 2 cups hot cooked quick-cooking brown rice mixed with ¼ cup chopped peanuts

COMPLETE MEAL SERVING
384 calories / 12 g total fat / 112 calories from fat / 29% calories from fat
65 mg cholesterol / 155 mg sodium / 37 g carbohydrate / 5 g fiber / 6 g sugars / 31 g protein

Orange Pork Saute

Prep Time: 10 minutes ■ Cook Time: 8 minutes

Quicker than delivery, this delicious pork dish features citrus juices flavored with zesty cumin and cilantro. If you're not a cilantro fan, go for fresh basil instead.

3	tablespoons all-purpose flour
1	teaspoon ground cumin
⅛	teaspoon ground black pepper
4	boneless lean pork cutlets (1 pound)
	Nonstick cooking spray
1	clove garlic, minced
½	cup orange juice
2	tablespoons lemon juice
2	tablespoons snipped fresh cilantro

1 In large resealable plastic bag combine flour, cumin, and pepper. Add pork and toss to coat.

2 In nonstick skillet lightly sprayed with nonstick cooking spray cook pork over medium heat for 6 minutes or until juices run clear, turning once. Place on serving plate; keep warm.

3 Add garlic to skillet and cook for 1 minute. Add orange juice and lemon juice and cook for 1 minute or until slightly thickened. Pour sauce over pork and sprinkle with cilantro.

Makes 4 servings

to complete the meal For 4 servings: 3 cups hot cooked wild rice ■ 1 large bunch broccoli, steamed

COMPLETE MEAL SERVING
449 calories / 13 g total fat / 118 calories from fat / 26% calories from fat
101 mg cholesterol / 124 mg sodium / 43 g carbohydrate / 7 g fiber / 7 g sugars / 42 g protein

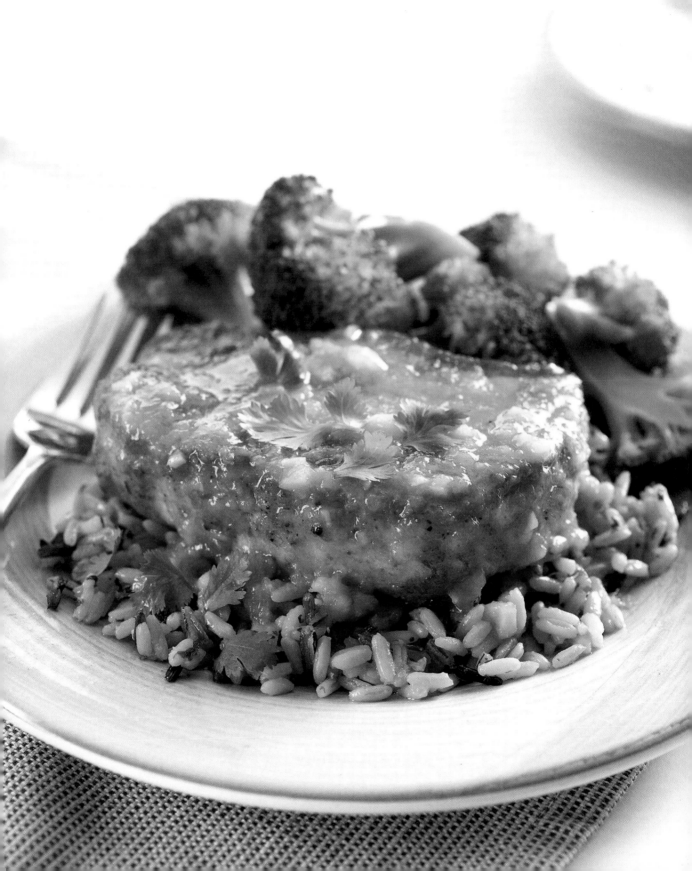

Pork Chops with Pear Sauce

Prep Time: 10 minutes ■ Cook Time: 17 minutes

Pears are the one fruit best picked before ripening. Select pears with smooth skins without blemishes. Ripen the pears at room temperature in a paper bag.

4	bone-in pork loin chops (about 2 pounds), trimmed of visible fat
½	teaspoon salt
⅛	teaspoon ground black pepper
	Nonstick cooking spray
2	cups chopped fennel (1) or celery
1	firm ripe pear, cored and cut into ½-inch pieces
½	tablespoon all-purpose flour
¾	cup apple juice
¼	cup dried cherries
1	tablespoon plus 1 teaspoon snipped fresh sage
1	tablespoon minced crystallized ginger or ½ teaspoon dried ginger

1 Season pork with salt and pepper.

2 In large skillet lightly sprayed with nonstick cooking spray cook pork over medium heat for 6 minutes or until brown, turning once. Remove to plate.

3 Add fennel and cook for 3 minutes, stirring occasionally. Add pear and cook for 2 minutes. Stir in flour and cook for 1 minute. Stir in apple juice, cherries, sage, and ginger.

4 Bring to boiling over high heat. Return pork and any juices to skillet. Reduce heat to medium-low; cover and cook for 5 minutes or until meat thermometer registers 160°F and juices run clear.

Makes 4 servings

to complete the meal For 4 servings: 2 cups hot cooked orzo tossed with ¼ cup grated Parmesan cheese and 1 teaspoon trans-fat-free canola margarine ■ 1 pound asparagus, steamed

COMPLETE MEAL SERVING
451 calories / 13 g total fat / 113 calories from fat / 25% calories from fat
96 mg cholesterol / 491 mg sodium / 43 g carbohydrate / 4 g fiber / 17 g sugars / 41 g protein

Baked Pork Chops and Rice

Prep Time: 10 minutes ■ Cook Time: 1 hour

Healthful brown rice differs from white rice in that the bran has not been removed. The bran contains most of the fiber and nutrients, so switching from white to brown rice is a great decision for good health.

	Nonstick cooking spray
4	bone-in center-cut pork loin chops (about 2 pounds), trimmed
2¼	teaspoons curry powder
1	cup chopped onion (1 large)
1	cup uncooked brown rice
2½	cups fat-free chicken broth
½	cup chopped dried fruit
1	tablespoon plus 1 teaspoon ginger marinade
¼	cup snipped fresh cilantro

1 Preheat oven to 350°F. Lightly spray 13×9-inch baking pan with nonstick cooking spray.

2 Rub both sides of pork with curry powder.

3 In large nonstick skillet lightly sprayed with nonstick cooking spray cook pork over medium-high heat for 4 minutes or until brown, turning once. Remove to plate.

4 In same skillet cook and stir onion over medium heat for 3 minutes. Add rice, stirring to coat with oil. Stir in broth, dried fruit, and marinade. Bring to boiling over high heat.

5 Place rice mixture into prepared pan. Arrange pork on top of rice mixture. Cover tightly with foil and bake for 45 minutes or until rice is tender and meat thermometer registers 160°F in pork and juices run clear. Stir in cilantro before serving.

Makes 4 servings

to complete the meal   For 4 servings: 1 cup sliced avocado and 1 sliced tomato

COMPLETE MEAL SERVING
561 calories / 17 g total fat / 154 calories from fat / 27% calories from fat
98 mg cholesterol / 720 mg sodium / 58 g carbohydrate / 7 g fiber / 17 g sugars / 43 g protein

Pork Chops with Watermelon Salsa

Prep Time: 20 minutes ■ Cook Time: 8 minutes

Jicama, sometimes called a Mexican potato, is a large bulbous root with tan skin that should be peeled before using. Its nutty, sweet flavor and crunchy texture are perfect for salads, salsas, and snack sticks.

4   bone-in lean pork rib chops (about 1½ pounds)

1   tablespoon ancho chile powder

3   cups watermelon (about 2 pounds), cut into ½-inch pieces

1⅓   cups jicama, peeled and cut into ½-inch pieces

2   tablespoons snipped fresh cilantro

1   tablespoon minced jalapeño pepper (see tip, page 34)

1   tablespoon lime juice

    Nonstick cooking spray

½   cup diced avocado

1 Rub both sides of pork with chile powder; set aside

2 In large bowl combine watermelon, jicama, cilantro, jalapeño, and lime juice. Toss to coat.

3 In large skillet lightly sprayed with nonstick cooking spray cook pork over medium heat for 8 minutes or until meat thermometer registers 160°F and juices run clear, turning once.

4 Garnish each pork chop with watermelon salsa and avocado.

Makes 4 servings

to complete the meal   For 4 servings: 2 cups hot cooked quick-cooking brown rice ■ 4 fresh or frozen medium ears corn on the cob, cooked, and topped with 2 teaspoons trans-fat-free canola margarine

COMPLETE MEAL SERVING
386 calories / 12 g total fat / 107 calories from fat / 26% calories from fat
69 mg cholesterol / 97 mg sodium / 45 g carbohydrate / 8 g fiber / 16 g sugars / 31 g protein

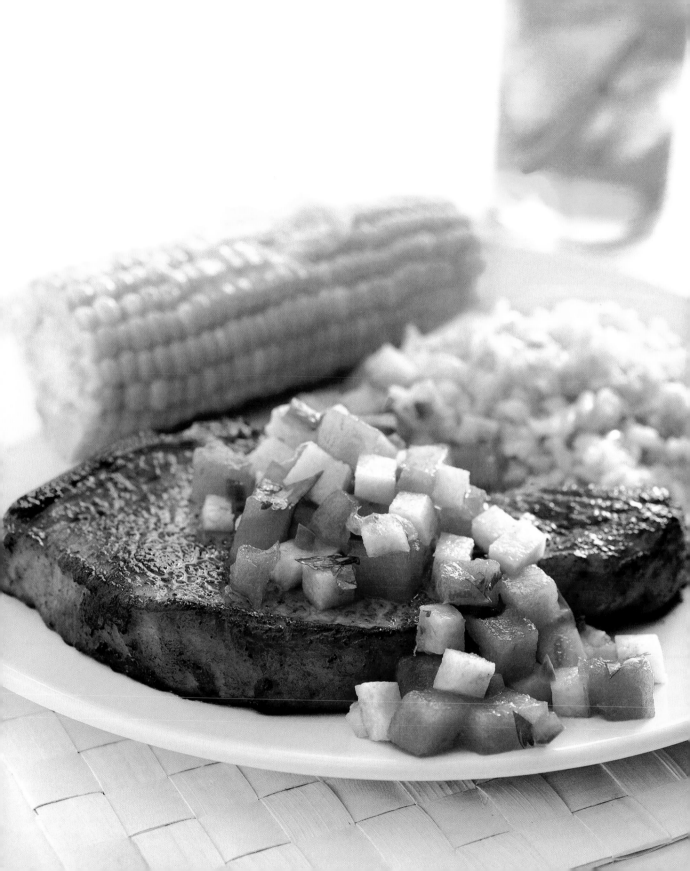

Pork Medallions with Garlicky Greens

Prep Time: 10 minutes ■ Cook Time: 16 minutes

For speedy meal preparation, keep jars of chopped ginger and chopped garlic in the refrigerator. Simply remove 1 teaspoon of garlic per clove required. Use the same amount of chopped ginger as called for in the recipe.

Nonstick cooking spray
2 tablespoons minced fresh ginger
4 6-ounce boneless center-cut pork loin chops
2 large cloves garlic, minced
4 cups torn romaine lettuce
2 cups watercress (tough stems removed)
3 cups packed baby spinach leaves (about 4½ ounces)
1 tablespoon low-sodium soy sauce

1 In large skillet lightly sprayed with nonstick cooking spray cook 1 tablespoon ginger over medium heat for 1 minute, stirring occasionally. Add pork and cook for 8 minutes or until meat thermometer registers 160°F and juices run clear. Remove pork to plate; keep warm.

2 In same skillet cook the remaining 1 tablespoon ginger and garlic for 2 minutes. Increase heat to medium-high; cook romaine, watercress, and spinach for 3 minutes or until greens wilt, stirring frequently. Stir in soy sauce; cook for 2 minutes, stirring frequently. Return pork and any juices to skillet; heat through.

Makes 4 servings

to complete the meal For 4 servings: 2 cups hot cooked orzo sprinkled with 2 tablespoons toasted sesame seeds ■ 1 pound peeled baby carrots, steamed

COMPLETE MEAL SERVING
418 calories / 12 g total fat / 110 calories from fat / 27% calories from fat
100 mg cholesterol / 327 mg sodium / 34 g carbohydrate / 6 g fiber / 8 g sugars / 42 g protein

Pork-Red Onion Kabobs

Prep Time: 20 minutes ■ Cook Time: 5 minutes

Although it's a summer squash, zucchini is available year-round. Select ones with smooth, blemish-free skin that are not too large, about 12 ounces. They will be tender and flavorful.

2	tablespoons lemon juice
1	teaspoon dried oregano, crushed
⅛	teaspoon ground black pepper
1½	pounds lean boneless pork loin, cut into twenty-four 1½-inch pieces
1	large red onion, quartered
2	medium zucchini, halved and cut into 1-inch slices

1 Preheat broiler.

2 In large bowl whisk together lemon juice, oregano, and pepper. Add pork, onion, and zucchini; toss to coat. Let stand for 10 minutes.

3 Alternately thread pork, onion, and zucchini onto four 12-inch metal skewers.

4 Broil 5 inches from heat for 5 minutes or until pork is no longer pink and vegetables are brown, turning once.

Makes 4 servings

to complete the meal   For 4 servings: 2 cups hot cooked jasmine rice ■ 4 tomatoes, sliced and drizzled with ½ cup fat-free Italian dressing and ½ cup reduced-fat shredded mozzarella

COMPLETE MEAL SERVING
474 calories / 14 g total fat / 124 calories from fat / 27% calories from fat
100 mg cholesterol / 468 mg sodium / 42 g carbohydrate / 4 g fiber / 9 g sugars / 42 g protein

moving forward
Bake, roast, grill, or broil your food instead of frying.

Ham Steaks with Fruit Salsa

Prep Time: 18 minutes ■ Cook Time: 5 minutes

Cilantro, sometimes called Chinese parsley or coriander, is the leaves and stems of the coriander plant. Its pungent flavor characterizes Mexican, Caribbean, and Asian cooking. You can substitute parsley if you prefer a milder flavor.

4	tablespoons apricot jam
1	tablespoon jalapeño pepper sauce
1	cup chopped mango (1)
2	cups chopped honeydew melon
¾	cup chopped seedless cucumber
¼	cup snipped fresh cilantro
2	tablespoons chopped green onion (1)
¼	cup pecans
	Nonstick cooking spray
1	12-ounce boneless low-sodium ham steak

1 In medium bowl stir together jam and jalapeño sauce until combined. Remove 2 tablespoons to small dish and set aside. Add mango, honeydew, cucumber, cilantro, green onion, and pecans to bowl; toss to coat.

2 In large skillet lightly sprayed with nonstick cooking spray cook ham over medium-high heat for 5 minutes or until heated through, turning once. Remove to plate and drizzle with reserved jam mixture. Serve with salsa.

Makes 4 servings

to complete the meal   Per serving: 1 medium sweet potato, baked, with 1 tablespoon sour cream

COMPLETE MEAL SERVING
433 calories / 14 g total fat / 121 calories from fat / 27% calories from fat
51 mg cholesterol / 884 mg sodium / 59 g carbohydrate / 6 g fiber / 39 g sugars / 22 g protein

Ham and Split Pea Chowder

Prep Time: 20 minutes ■ Cook Time: 8 to 10 hours (low), 4 to 6 hours (high)

This recipe makes a hearty, chunky chowder. For a supervelvety texture, puree the mixture using an immersion blender or in batches with a standard blender before adding the remaining ham.

	Nonstick cooking spray
1¼	pounds low-sodium extra lean ham (5% fat), cut into ½-inch cubes
1	pound dried split peas, rinsed and picked over
1	cup chopped onion (1 large)
1	cup chopped celery (2 stalks)
1	pound baby carrots, sliced
1	teaspoon dried thyme, crushed
¼	teaspoon crushed red pepper flakes
2	14½-ounce cans fat-free low-sodium chicken broth
3	cups water

1 In large skillet lightly sprayed with nonstick cooking spray cook and stir ham over medium heat for 5 minutes or until brown. Remove half the ham to bowl; cover and refrigerate.

2 In a 5- to 6-quart slow cooker layer split peas, onion, celery, carrot, thyme, and pepper flakes. Top with broth, the water, and the remaining ham.

3 Cover and cook on low-heat setting for 8 to 10 hours or on high-heat setting for 4 to 6 hours or until peas have dissolved and vegetables are fork-tender. Stir in remaining refrigerated ham and let stand 5 minutes or until ham is heated through.

Makes 8 servings

to complete the meal For 8 servings: 8 cups torn romaine lettuce leaves tossed with 1 cup toasted pine nuts, ½ cup fat-free balsamic vinaigrette, and 2 tablespoons artificial bacon bits

COMPLETE MEAL SERVING
417 calories / 12 g total fat / 109 calories from fat / 25% calories from fat
30 mg cholesterol / 867 mg sodium / 50 g carbohydrate / 15 g fiber / 14 g sugars / 32 g protein

Peppered Beef Tenderloin

Prep Time: 5 minutes n Cook Time: 1 hour

Meat roasts, whether beef or pork, should always stand for 10 minutes before slicing. The meat will continue cooking, allowing the roast to come to the optimal temperature, but it also allows for the natural juices to seep back into the center of the roast.

1 3-pound lean beef tenderloin roast (large end), trimmed of visible fat
2 tablespoons peppercorn mélange blend of black, red, green, and white peppercorns
2 cloves garlic, minced
¾ teaspoon salt

1 Preheat oven to 450°F.

2 Place beef on rack in large roasting pan.

3 Place peppercorns in small resealable plastic bag; seal, removing all air from bag. Using rolling pin or heavy skillet, crush peppercorns. Add garlic and salt to bag, shaking to blend. Rub peppercorn mixture over beef, pressing to adhere.

4 Roast for 1 hour for medium rare or until meat thermometer registers 135°F. Cover with foil; let stand 10 minutes. Temperature of meat after standing should be 145°F.

Makes 8 servings

to complete the meal   For 8 servings: 3 pounds red potatoes, quartered, cooked in boiling water until tender, and mashed with ⅓ cup reduced-fat buttermilk and ¼ cup shredded reduced-fat cheddar cheese ■ 2 medium (12-ounce) zucchini, quartered and sliced into ½-inch pieces and steamed

COMPLETE MEAL SERVING
398 calories / 12 g total fat / 104 calories from fat / 25% calories from fat
88 mg cholesterol / 188 mg sodium / 38 g carbohydrate / 5 g fiber / 5 g sugars / 35 g protein

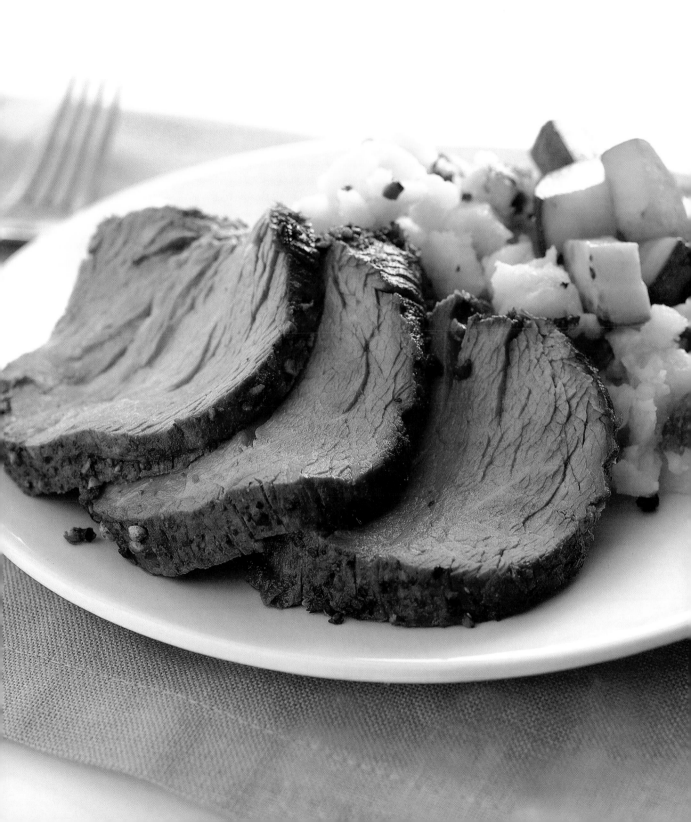

Grilled Flank Steak

Prep Time: 10 minutes ■ Cook Time: 12 minutes

You don't often think of using maple syrup on steak, but here the syrup combines with mustard, tomato paste, and vinegar for a delicious tangy sauce. There's plenty of sauce to eat with the steak and a bit to mop up with the roasted potatoes. Yum!

Nonstick grilling spray
1 2½-pound flank steak
¼ teaspoon salt
¼ teaspoon ground black pepper
¼ cup finely chopped shallot (1 large)
2 cloves garlic, finely chopped
⅓ cup maple syrup
⅓ cup red wine vinegar
¼ cup country-style Dijon mustard
2 tablespoons tomato paste
2 teaspoons Worcestershire sauce

1 Lightly spray grill grate with nonstick grilling spray and heat to medium-high.

2 Season both sides of steak with salt and pepper. Grill steak for 12 minutes or until medium doneness (160°F), turning once. Remove steak from grill and cover loosely with foil; let stand 10 minutes.

3 Meanwhile, in small saucepan lightly sprayed with nonstick cooking spray cook and stir shallot for 2 minutes or until tender and golden brown. Add garlic; cook and stir 1 minute. Add maple syrup, vinegar, mustard, tomato paste, and Worcestershire; bring to boiling. Remove from heat and keep warm.

4 To serve, slice steak diagonally across the grain and serve with warm sauce.

Makes 8 servings

to complete the meal For 8 servings: 3 pounds red potatoes, halved, lightly sprayed with nonstick cooking spray, roasted, and topped with 1 teaspoon trans-fat-free canola margarine per serving ■ 8 cups mesclun tossed with 1 large yellow sweet pepper, cut into ½-inch strips, and 1 chopped tomato and drizzled with ½ cup fat-free red wine vinaigrette

COMPLETE MEAL SERVING
465 calories / 13 g total fat / 120 calories from fat / 26% calories from fat
68 mg cholesterol / 462 mg sodium / 52 g carbohydrate / 5 g fiber / 14 g sugars / 33 g protein

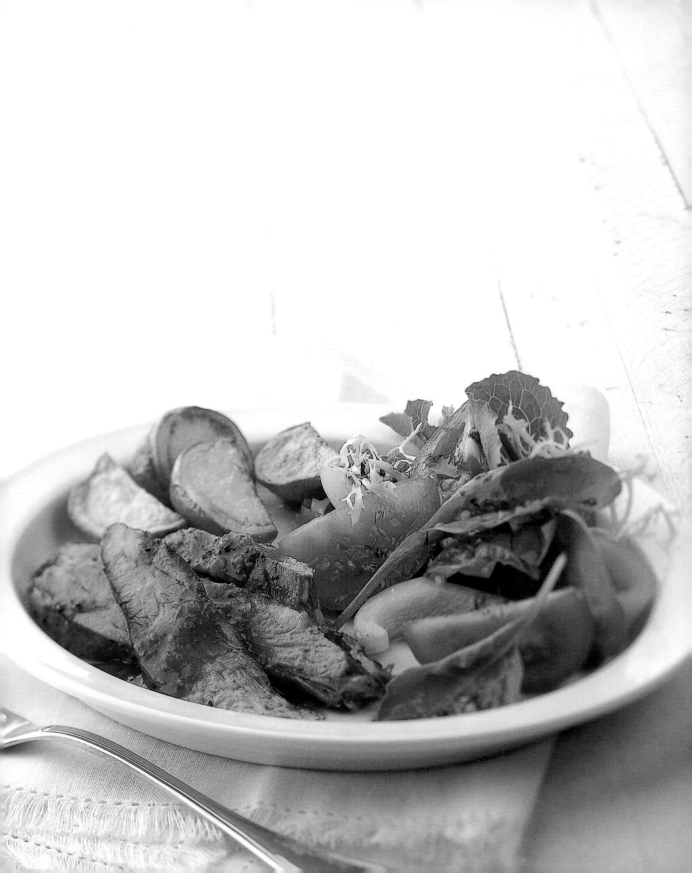

Sirloin with Mushroom Sauce

Prep Time: 10 minutes ■ Cook Time: 15 minutes

Shiitake mushrooms, which are known for their immune-boosting properties, add an earthy, smoky flavor to dishes. They're available both fresh and dried, although the dried ones need to be rehydrated and are best in soups, stews, and stir-fries.

1	1½-pound boneless lean sirloin steak
4	cups sliced assorted mushrooms, such as shiitake, cremini, and baby bella
2	shallots, sliced
2	cloves garlic, finely chopped
3	tablespoons balsamic vinegar
1	tablespoon Dijon mustard
¼	teaspoon ground black pepper
¾	cup reduced-sodium beef broth

1 Preheat broiler.

2 Place steak in bottom of broiler pan. Arrange mushrooms, shallot, and garlic around steak in pan.

3 In medium bowl whisk together vinegar, mustard, and pepper. Drizzle half of dressing over steak and mushrooms.

4 Broil steak and mushrooms 3 inches from heat for 6 minutes. Turn steak, stir mushrooms, and drizzle both with remaining dressing. Broil for 6 minutes for medium rare (145°F). Remove steak to cutting board; let stand for 10 minutes. Stir broth into pan and broil for 3 minutes.

5 To serve, thinly slice steak diagonally across the grain. Serve topped with mushroom sauce.

Makes 4 servings

to complete the meal For 4 servings: 1½ pounds yellow-flesh potatoes mashed with ½ cup low-fat buttermilk and ¾ cup shredded reduced-fat cheddar cheese
■ one 10-ounce box frozen green peas, steamed

COMPLETE MEAL SERVING
528 calories / 14 g total fat / 130 calories from fat / 25% calories from fat
111 mg cholesterol / 307 mg sodium / 49 g carbohydrate / 6 g fiber / 8 g sugars / 50 g protein

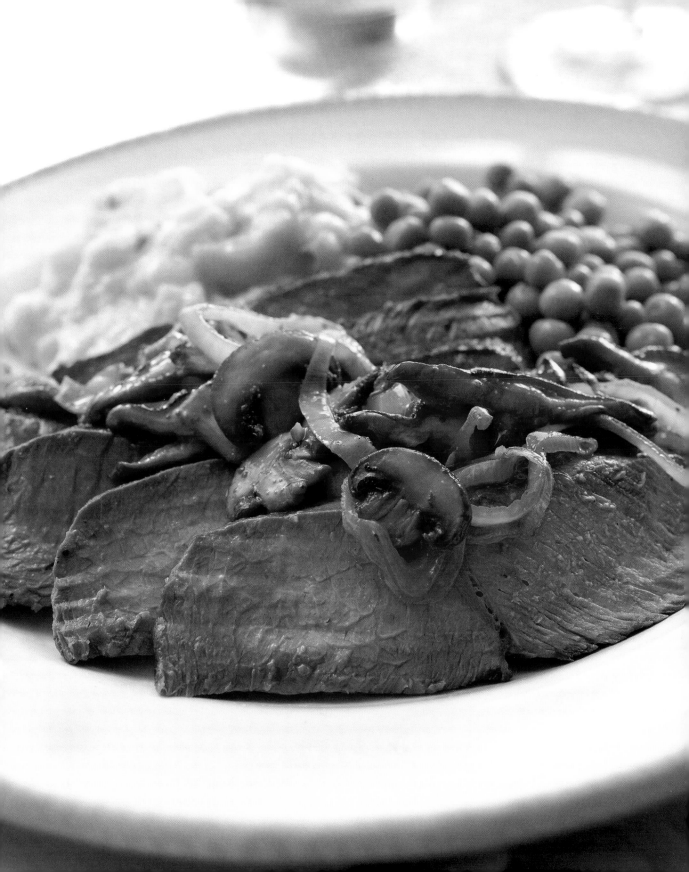

Oven-Braised Beef Brisket

Prep Time: 5 minutes ■ Cook Time: 3 hours, 10 minutes

When selecting beef for this or any recipe, choose beef with a bright cherry red color without any grayish or brown blotches. A darker purplish red color is typical of vacuum-packaged beef. Be sure the packages are cold, tightly wrapped, and have no tears or punctures. Steaks, roasts, and pot roasts should be firm to the touch, not soft.

1	3-pound boneless lean beef brisket, trimmed of visible fat
1	teaspoon garlic powder
½	teaspoon salt
½	teaspoon ground black pepper
	Nonstick cooking spray
1	14-ounce can reduced-sodium beef broth
¾	cup red wine
¼	cup orange juice
⅓	cup packed brown sugar

1 Preheat oven to 325°F.

2 Season brisket with garlic powder, salt, and pepper.

3 In deep-dish ovenproof skillet or Dutch oven lightly sprayed with nonstick cooking spray cook brisket over medium-high heat for 8 minutes, turning to brown on all sides. Remove brisket from skillet. Add broth, wine, orange juice, and brown sugar to skillet. Bring to boiling, scraping brown bits from bottom of pan. Remove from heat and return brisket to pan.

4 Cover and bake for 3 hours or until brisket is very tender.

Makes 12 servings

to complete the meal   For 12 servings: 3 pounds red potatoes quartered, lightly sprayed with nonstick cooking spray and roasted ■ 2 pounds green beans, steamed, and ¾ cup sliced almonds ■ twelve 1-ounce whole wheat rolls each spread with ½ teaspoon trans-fat-free canola margarine

COMPLETE MEAL SERVING
406 calories/ 13 g total fat / 113 calories from fat / 27% calories from fat
48 mg cholesterol / 320 mg sodium / 51 g carbohydrate / 7 g fiber / 12 g sugars / 25 g protein

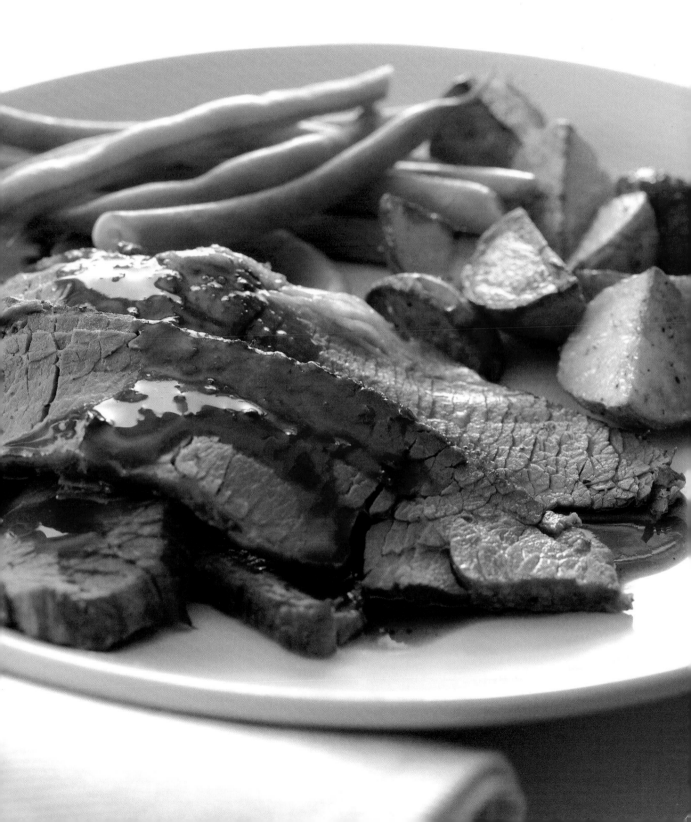

Spinach-Stuffed Steak

Prep Time: 20 minutes ■ Cook Time: 14 minutes

If spinach reminds you only of Popeye, give this brilliant green vegetable a second thought. Packed with vitamins, minerals, and antioxidants, it's a nutritional powerhouse. When prepared in dishes like this one, its flavor mellows and blends beautifully with the meat, garlic, and sweet pepper.

1	cup chopped red sweet pepper (1 large)
2	cloves garlic, minced
1	teaspoon olive oil
4	cups packed baby spinach leaves
¼	cup grated low-fat Parmesan cheese
1	1-pound beef top round steak, ¾ inch thick
2	teaspoons spicy steak seasoning
2	red onions, cut into thin wedges

1 Preheat broiler.

2 In large nonstick skillet cook and stir sweet pepper and garlic in hot oil over medium heat for 3 minutes or until light brown. Increase heat to medium-high. Add spinach; cook for 3 minutes or until spinach wilts, stirring frequently. Remove spinach mixture to large metal bowl or baking pan. Place in freezer to cool down quickly. Stir in cheese.

3 Meanwhile, place steak on work surface. Using sharp knife, cut large pocket into side of steak. Fill pocket with spinach mixture. Rub both sides of the steak with steak seasoning. Place steak on rack in broiler pan with onion wedges. Broil steak and onion 3 inches from heat for 8 minutes for medium rare (145°F), turning once. Place steak and onion wedges on serving platter. Let steak stand 5 minutes before slicing.

Makes 4 servings

to complete the meal For 4 servings: one 20-ounce bag frozen crispy waffle fries, baked

COMPLETE MEAL SERVING
458 calories / 15 g total fat / 135 calories from fat / 29% calories from fat
53 mg cholesterol / 585 mg sodium / 48 g carbohydrate / 6 g fiber / 4 g sugars / 32 g protein

Thai-Style Beef Tacos

Prep Time: 18 minutes ■ Cook Time: 12 minutes

Delicious flavor combinations like this have made it possible to eat healthfully without straying off track. Don't be put off by the fish sauce. Think of it as salt. It's an outrageously delicious high-impact, zero-calorie flavor ingredient.

¼ cup lime juice
1 tablespoon finely minced shallot
  Nonstick grilling spray
¾ pound flank steak
½ teaspoon ground black pepper
¼ cup snipped fresh cilantro
2 tablespoons fish sauce
2 teaspoons sugar
1 teaspoon Vietnamese chili paste
1 cucumber, peeled, halved, seeded, and thinly sliced
1 mango, peeled, seeded, and cut into 1-inch chunks
4 cups watermelon chunks
12 6-inch corn tortillas
¾ cup low-fat sour cream

1 In large bowl pour ¼ cup of the lime juice over shallot; let stand.

2 Lightly spray grill grate with nonstick grilling spray and heat to medium-high.

3 Season steak with pepper. Grill steak for 12 minutes or until medium doneness (160°F), turning once. Remove steak from grill and cover loosely with foil; let stand 10 minutes. Thinly slice.

4 To bowl with shallot add cilantro, fish sauce, sugar, and chili paste. Stir until sugar dissolves. Add cucumber, mango, and watermelon; toss to coat.

5 Divide tortillas among 4 plates. Divide salad and steak on tortillas. Top each tortilla with 3 tablespoons of the sour cream.

Makes 4 servings

COMPLETE MEAL SERVING
506 calories / 16 g total fat / 146 calories from fat / 29% calories from fat
60 mg cholesterol / 861 mg sodium / 69 g carbohydrate / 8 g fiber / 27 g sugars / 26 g protein

Steaks with Yogurt Sauce

Prep Time: 10 minutes ■ Cook Time: 8 minutes

Dry rub, a blend of spices or herbs, salt, and pepper, imparts flavor into meats. The mixture can be rubbed onto the meat just before cooking, or for a more pronounced flavor, the meat with dry rub can be lightly wrapped in plastic wrap and refrigerated for up to 24 hours.

4	6-ounce beef eye round steaks, ½ inch thick
2	teaspoons ground cumin
¼	teaspoon ground black pepper
1	cup plain low-fat yogurt
1	cup finely chopped, peeled and seeded cucumber
2	tablespoons snipped fresh cilantro
1	clove garlic, minced
	Nonstick cooking spray
2	tomatoes, cored and cut into ½-inch slices
⅓	cup chopped peanuts

1 Rub steaks with cumin and pepper; set aside for 10 minutes.

2 In medium bowl combine yogurt, cucumber, cilantro, and garlic; toss to coat.

3 In large skillet lightly sprayed with nonstick cooking spray cook tomato over medium heat for 3 minutes or until brown, turning once. Remove to serving plate.

4 In same skillet cook steaks over medium-high heat for 5 minutes, turning once for medium rare (145°F). Serve steaks with tomato, sauce, and peanuts.

Makes 4 servings

to complete the meal   Per serving: one 6½-inch whole wheat pita

COMPLETE MEAL SERVING
509 calories / 15 g total fat / 131 calories from fat / 25% calories from fat
91 mg cholesterol / 473 mg sodium / 47 g carbohydrate / 7 g fiber / 8 g sugars / 50 g protein

Marinated Tenderloin in Chipotle Sauce

Prep Time: 10 minutes ■ Cook Time: 10 minutes

Delicious chunks of lean beef bathed in a smoky chipotle sauce and seared with aromatic vegetables add up to a dish bursting with flavor that's ready in less than 30 minutes! Special enough for guests, this colorful dish is a winner.

1½	pounds lean beef tenderloin or sirloin, cubed
¼	cup chipotle pepper sauce
	Nonstick cooking spray
1	cup chopped onion (1 large)
3	cloves garlic, chopped
1	14½-ounce can diced tomatoes, drained
1	large green sweet pepper, cut into ½-inch strips

1 In medium bowl combine beef and chipotle sauce; set aside.

2 In large skillet lightly sprayed with nonstick cooking spray cook onion, garlic, and tomatoes over medium-high heat for 5 minutes or until onion is tender.

3 Add marinated beef and sweet pepper; cook and stir for 5 minutes or until beef is slightly pink in center.

Makes 6 servings

to complete the meal For 6 servings: 3 cups hot cooked white rice tossed with ¼ cup snipped fresh cilantro ■ 1 bunch broccoli, steamed

COMPLETE MEAL SERVING
388 calories / 12 g total fat / 107 calories from fat / 28% calories from fat
95 mg cholesterol / 230 mg sodium / 32 g carbohydrate / 5 g fiber / 8 g sugars / 38 g protein

Vegetable-Beef Stir-Fry

Prep Time: 3 minutes ■ Cook Time: 8 minutes

Marry a stir-fry sauce with a fresh or frozen vegetable medley and lean protein for a delicious quick meal. To slice the steak easily, freeze the meat for 30 minutes, then slice.

Nonstick cooking spray
1 ¾-pound flank or sirloin steak, sliced very thin
½ cup Szechwan stir-fry sauce
¼ cup water
1 1½-pound bag frozen vegetable medley mix, thawed

1 In large skillet lightly sprayed with nonstick cooking spray cook steak over medium-high heat for 5 minutes or until meat is cooked to your preference, stirring constantly. Place on plate.

2 Add sauce and the water to the skillet; bring to a simmer. Reduce heat to medium, add vegetables, and cook for 2 minutes or until heated through. Return meat to skillet; cook for 1 minute.

Makes 4 servings

to complete the meal For 4 servings: 3 cups hot cooked quick-cooking brown rice, mixed with ¼ cup dry-roasted cashews

COMPLETE MEAL SERVING
429 calories / 12 g total fat / 112 calories from fat / 27% calories from fat
36 mg cholesterol / 214 mg sodium / 53 g carbohydrate / 7 g fiber / 8 g sugars / 23 g protein

moving forward
Emphasize your good work and each new goal you meet by treating yourself.

Beef and Barley Stew

Prep Time: 20 minutes ■ Cook Time: 8 to 10 hours (low), 4 to 6 hours (high)

If time permits and you'd like to add a nutty flavor to the barley, toast it before adding to the slow cooker. To toast barley or any whole grain, place it in a nonstick skillet over medium heat. Cook the grain while stirring occasionally for 3 minutes or until light brown.

	Nonstick cooking spray
1	pound cubed boneless beef chuck
2	cups water
2	cups chopped onion (2 medium)
12	ounces parsnips, sliced (2 cups)
1½	cups sliced baby carrot
1	10-ounce package sliced mushrooms, halved
1	cup uncooked pearl barley
2	teaspoons Italian seasoning
2	14½-ounce cans reduced-sodium beef broth

1 In large nonstick skillet lightly sprayed with nonstick cooking spray cook half of the beef over medium-high heat for 5 minutes, turning to brown all sides. Place in 3½- or 4-quart slow cooker. Repeat with remaining beef. Add the water to skillet, stirring to scrape brown bits from bottom. Remove from heat and add to slow cooker with onion, parsnip, carrot, mushrooms, barley, and Italian seasoning. Pour broth over mixture.

2 Cover and cook for 8 to 10 hours on low-heat setting or 4 to 6 hours on high-heat setting until beef and vegetables are fork-tender.

Makes 6 servings

to complete the meal   Per serving: one 1½-ounce seven-grain roll, 1 teaspoon
trans-fat-free canola margarine

COMPLETE MEAL SERVING
453 calories / 14 g total fat / 121 calories from fat / 26% calories from fat
52 mg cholesterol / 338 mg sodium / 57 g carbohydrate / 10 g fiber / 10 g sugars / 28 g protein

Hearty Beef Stew

Prep Time: 5 minutes ■ Cook Time: 1 hour 37 minutes

Italian seasoning is a dried herb mixture usually containing marjoram, thyme, rosemary, savory, sage, oregano, and basil. Look for it in the spice and dried herb section of supermarkets. However, you can substitute a mixture of any of those herbs for the Italian seasoning.

1½	pounds lean beef stew meat, cut into 1- to 1½-inch pieces
3	tablespoons all-purpose flour
	Nonstick cooking spray
2	cloves garlic, minced
2	14½-ounce cans reduced-sodium beef broth
2	cups water
1	14½-ounce can no-salt-added diced tomatoes, undrained
¾	cup red wine
1	pound potatoes, peeled and cut into 1-inch pieces
2	cups baby carrots
2	cups frozen pearl onions
2	teaspoons Italian seasoning
1	tablespoon snipped fresh parsley

1 Place beef in resealable plastic bag. Add flour and gently shake to evenly coat beef with flour.

2 In Dutch oven or large stockpot lightly sprayed with nonstick cooking spray cook and stir half of the beef over medium-high heat for 3 minutes or until brown. Remove to bowl. Cook and stir remaining beef for 3 minutes or until brown. Place in bowl.

3 Add garlic to Dutch oven or stockpot; cook and stir for 1 minute. Add broth, the water, tomatoes, wine, potato, carrots, onions, and Italian seasoning. Bring to boiling; reduce heat, cover, and simmer for 1½ hours or until beef is tender. Divide among 4 bowls and garnish with parsley.

Makes 4 servings

COMPLETE MEAL SERVING
465 calories / 13 g total fat / 119 calories from fat / 26% calories from fat
106 mg cholesterol / 233 mg sodium / 44 g carbohydrate / 6 g fiber / 13 g sugars / 42 g protein

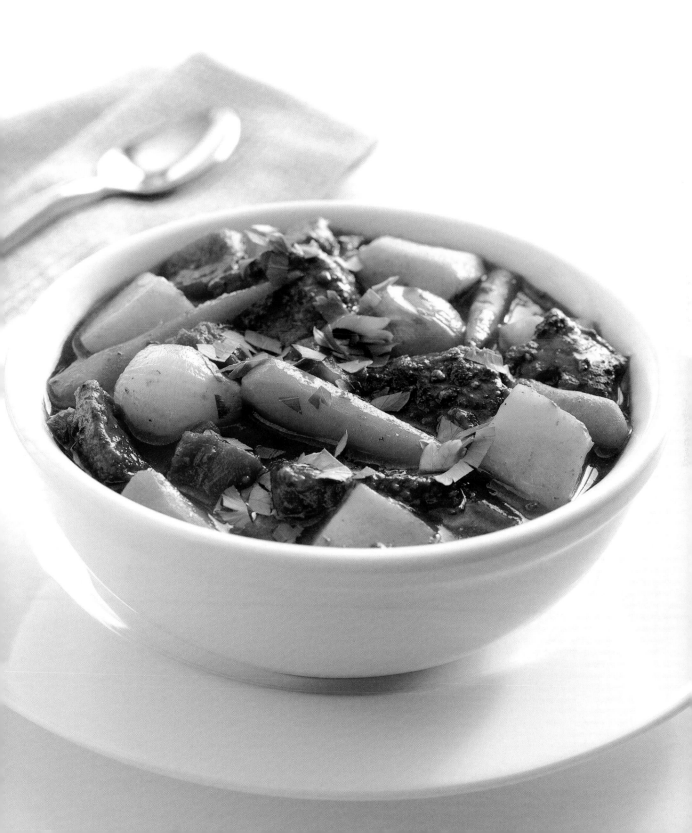

Cuban Meatball Kabobs

Prep Time: 10 minutes ■ Cook Time: 10 minutes

Adding fresh mango and cilantro to jarred salsa heightens the flavor with a sweet, fresh twist. It's delicious served on top of zesty meatballs.

1	cup mild chunky salsa
1	medium ripe mango, peeled, seeded, and cubed
2	tablespoons snipped fresh cilantro
¾	pound lean ground beef
1	cup chopped red onion (1 large)
¾	cup quick-cooking rolled oats
¼	cup fat-free (skim) milk
3	cloves garlic, minced
¼	cup snipped fresh cilantro
1	teaspoon dried oregano, crushed
½	teaspoon ground cumin
4	6-inch corn tortillas, warmed

1 Preheat broiler.

2 In medium bowl combine salsa, mango, and 2 tablespoons cilantro; set aside.

3 In large bowl combine beef, onion, oats, milk, garlic, ¼ cup cilantro, oregano, and cumin. Shape into 12 balls and divide among 4 metal skewers.

4 Place skewers on rack in broiling pan. Broil 3 inches from heat for 10 minutes or until meat thermometer inserted into meatballs registers 160°F, turning once.

5 Place 1 tortilla on each of 4 plates. Remove meatballs from skewers and divide meatballs and salsa among tortillas.

Makes 4 servings

to complete the meal　For 4 servings: 6 cups torn romaine lettuce, 1 diced tomato, and 1 cup diced avocado tossed with ½ cup fat-free balsamic vinaigrette

COMPLETE MEAL SERVING
407 calories / 14 g total fat / 126 calories from fat / 30% calories from fat
24 mg cholesterol / 678 mg sodium / 53 g carbohydrate / 9 g fiber / 18 g sugars / 21 g protein

Grandma's Pot Roast

Prep Time: 10 minutes ■ Cook Time: 6 to 8 hours (low), 3 to 4 hours (high)

Here's a great meal that prepares itself while you're out for the day. Combine the wine, ketchup, and gravy mix in a small jar, shake to blend, and refrigerate the night before. The next morning, simply shake to blend the gravy mixture, pour it around the vegetables and roast, cover, set temperature, and be off.

1	pound fingerling or small red potatoes
1	16-ounce package baby carrots
1	2½-pound bottom round beef roast
1	teaspoon dried rosemary, crushed
½	teaspoon ground black pepper
½	cup red wine
⅓	cup ketchup
1	0.87-ounce package brown gravy mix

1 Place potatoes and carrots in a 3½- to 4-quart slow cooker. Place roast on top of vegetables; sprinkle half of the rosemary and half of the pepper over roast.

2 In small bowl whisk together wine, ketchup, gravy mix, remaining rosemary, and remaining pepper. Pour around roast in slow cooker. Cover and cook 6 to 8 hours on low-heat setting or 3 to 4 hours on high-heat setting until meat and vegetables are fork-tender. Skim fat off juices and serve juices with roast and vegetables.

Makes 6 servings

to complete the meal   For 6 servings: six 1½-ounce seven-grain rolls ■ 6 cups salad greens tossed with ⅓ cup fat-free balsamic vinaigrette

COMPLETE MEAL SERVING
524 calories / 16 g total fat / 141 calories from fat / 26% calories from fat
116 mg cholesterol / 912 mg sodium / 56 g carbohydrate / 7 g fiber / 13 g sugars / 46 g protein

moving forward
Don't consider exercise lost time. Taking care of yourself should be a priority.

Veal Piccata

Prep Time: 5 minutes ■ Cook Time: 9 minutes

A classic Italian dish, veal piccata is lightly floured veal that's quickly sauteed then drizzled with a sauce made from the pan drippings, lemon juice, and capers. Stirring cold butter into the sauce thickens it slightly and adds a delicious richness.

3	tablespoons all-purpose flour
¼	teaspoon ground black pepper
1	pound thinly sliced boneless veal cutlets, about ¼ inch thick
	Nonstick cooking spray
⅓	cup dry white wine
⅓	cup fat-free, reduced-sodium chicken broth
1½	tablespoons lemon juice
1	tablespoon drained nonpareil (petite) capers
1	tablespoon trans-fat-free canola margarine

1 On shallow plate combine flour and pepper. Dredge veal in flour mixture, shaking off excess flour.

2 In large nonstick skillet lightly sprayed with nonstick cooking spray cook half the veal over medium-high heat for 3 minutes or until cooked through, turning once. Remove to plate; keep warm. Repeat with remaining veal.

3 Add wine, broth, lemon juice, and capers to skillet, stirring up any brown bits from bottom. Bring to boiling over high heat. Boil for 3 minutes or until reduced slightly. Remove skillet from heat; whisk in margarine. Pour sauce over veal.

Makes 4 servings

to complete the meal   For 4 servings: 4 cups hot cooked wild rice ■ 1 pound asparagus, steamed ■ four 2-ounce whole wheat rolls

COMPLETE MEAL SERVING
559 calories / 17 g total fat / 153 calories from fat / 27% calories from fat
74 mg cholesterol / 471 mg sodium / 72 g carbohydrate / 8 g fiber / 5 g sugars / 33 g protein

Grilled Boneless Leg of Lamb

Prep Time: 10 minutes ■ Cook Time: 20 minutes

Leg of lamb comes either bone-in or boneless. A boneless leg is either rolled and tied or butterflied. This cut is perfect for grilling because it is flat with an even thickness, allowing for even cooking. If you can't find one in your market, ask the butcher to bone and butterfly it for you.

	Nonstick grilling spray
8	cloves garlic, minced
¼	cup snipped fresh rosemary
¼	cup snipped fresh mint
1	teaspoon salt
½	teaspoon ground black pepper
1	3-pound boneless butterflied leg of lamb
3	tablespoons lemon juice

1 Lightly spray grill rack with nonstick grilling spray and heat grill to medium-high.

2 In small bowl combine garlic, rosemary, mint, salt, and pepper. With tip of small, sharp knife, cut ½-inch-deep slits all over lamb. Rub garlic mixture into slits and all over lamb. Run 3 long wooden skewers through lamb to form a semisolid piece of meat.

3 Grill lamb for 20 minutes or until meat thermometer inserted into center of roast registers 140°F (medium rare), turning once. Place on plate and sprinkle with lemon juice. Let stand 10 minutes before slicing.

Makes 12 servings

to complete the meal   For 12 servings: 4½ pounds small red potatoes, quartered, and 1 large onion, chopped, roasted with 1 teaspoon olive oil ■ 1 large head cauliflower, steamed and topped with ½ cup shredded reduced-fat cheddar cheese ■ twelve 1-ounce whole wheat rolls each spread with 1 teaspoon trans-fat-free canola margarine

COMPLETE MEAL SERVING
446 calories / 13 g total fat / 112 calories from fat / 25% calories from fat
68 mg cholesterol / 487 mg sodium / 54 g carbohydrate / 7 g fiber / 6 g sugars / 30 g protein

Easy Crab Cakes

Prep Time: 5 minutes ■ Cook Time: 12 minutes

This dish is so simple you'll have these delicious crab cakes on the table in less than 20 minutes. It's so elegant you'll want to serve them for company. When cooking, resist the urge to move the crab cakes around; turning them just once keeps them intact and forms a nice crust.

2	6½-ounce cans lump crabmeat, drained, flaked, and cartilage removed
1¼	cups plain low-sodium bread crumbs
1	cup chopped red sweet pepper (1 large)
¼	cup chopped green onion (2)
½	cup fat-free, reduced-sodium Thousand Island dressing
¼	teaspoon cayenne pepper
	Nonstick cooking spray
6	cups mixed salad greens
2	medium apples, cored and cut into ¼-inch slices
½	cup sliced green olives
1	large carrot, shredded
¼	cup fat-free balsamic vinaigrette
1	cup shredded reduced-fat cheddar cheese

1 Line baking sheet with parchment or waxed paper.

2 In bowl using a rubber spatula, gently combine crabmeat, bread crumbs, sweet pepper, green onion, dressing, and cayenne pepper. Form into eight 2-inch crab cakes. Place on prepared baking sheet.

3 In large skillet lightly sprayed with nonstick cooking spray cook half of the crab cakes over medium heat for 6 minutes or until golden and heated through, turning once. Remove to plate. Repeat with remaining crab cakes.

4 Meanwhile, on large serving plate combine greens, apple, olives, and carrot. Drizzle with vinaigrette. Sprinkle with cheese. Top with cooked crab cakes.

Makes 4 servings

to complete the meal Per serving: 1-ounce whole wheat dinner roll with ½ teaspoon trans-fat-free canola margarine

COMPLETE MEAL SERVING
430 calories / 13 g total fat / 116 calories from fat / 26% calories from fat
76 mg cholesterol / 983 mg sodium / 56 g carbohydrate / 8 g fiber / 22 g sugars / 26 g protein

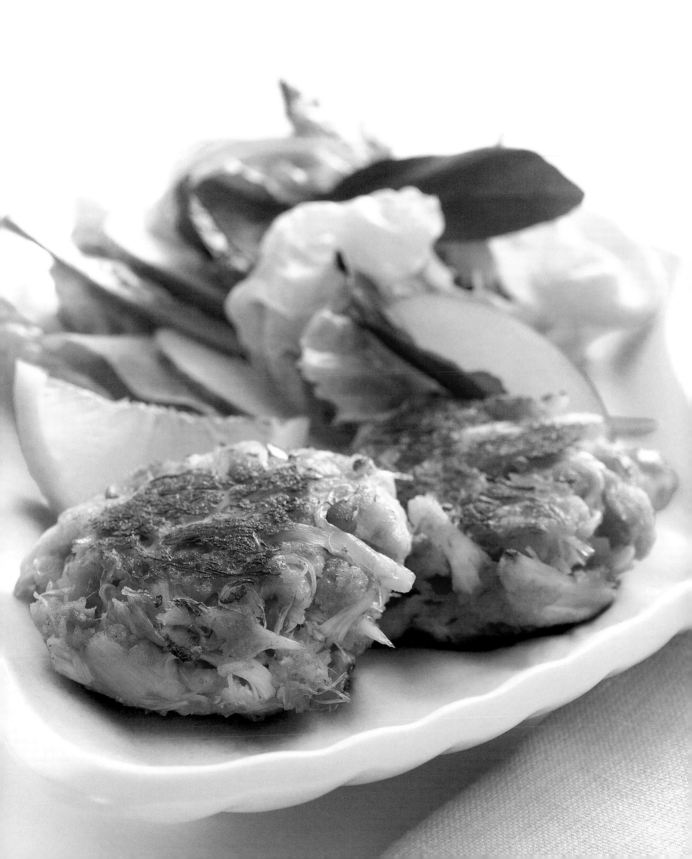

Hearty Manhattan Clam Chowder

Prep Time: 5 minutes ■ Cook Time: 25 minutes

Fennel, also known as sweet anise, has a bulbous base with celerylike stems and feathery fronds that are similar to dillweed. It has a mild licorice flavor. Chop or slice the bulb and stems as you would celery. Fennel adds a lovely flavor to salads, soups, and sautes.

¾	pound red potatoes, cut into ½-inch pieces
1	fennel bulb, trimmed and chopped
3	carrots, sliced lengthwise and bias-sliced
1	tablespoon dried Italian seasoning, crushed
1	teaspoon olive oil
2	14½-ounce cans no-salt-added diced tomatoes, undrained
½	cup canned unsalted corn kernels, drained
2	6½-ounce cans minced clams in juice, drained
½	cup grated Romano cheese

1 In Dutch oven or large stockpot cook potato, fennel, carrot, and Italian seasoning in hot oil over medium-high heat for 5 minutes or until vegetables are soft.

2 Add undrained tomatoes, corn, and clams. Cover and bring to boiling; reduce heat to medium and cook for 20 minutes or until potato is tender, stirring occasionally. Remove from heat and stir in cheese.

Makes 4 servings

to complete the meal Per serving: 1-ounce dinner roll with ½ teaspoon trans-fat-free canola margarine, 6 tablespoons toasted walnut halves

COMPLETE MEAL SERVING
398 calories / 12 g total fat / 111 calories from fat / 27% calories from fat
18 mg cholesterol / 867 mg sodium / 60 g carbohydrate / 12 g fiber / 14 g sugars / 17 g protein

moving forward
Shop for groceries after a meal. When you're hungry, foods look more tempting.

Fish Tacos with Salsa Verde

Prep Time: 10 minutes ■ Cook Time: 11 minutes

Mahi mahi, also known as dolphin or dorado, is not the lovely porpoises that perform at aquariums. It's a large fish with a firm white flesh and a mild flavor that is usually sold as fillets or steaks. It is available both fresh and frozen.

1	pound mahi mahi or other firm fish steak or fillet, cut into 1½-inch cubes
¼	cup snipped fresh cilantro
¼	cup chopped green onion (2)
2	tablespoons lime juice
	Nonstick grilling spray
1	pound tomatillos, husked and halved
	Nonstick cooking spray
4	whole wheat tortillas, warmed
¼	cup sour cream
½	cup chopped avocado

1 In medium bowl combine fish with 2 tablespoons of the cilantro, 2 tablespoons of the green onion, and lime juice; let marinate 10 minutes.

2 Meanwhile, lightly spray grill pan with nonstick grilling spray. Heat grill pan to high heat.

3 Lightly spray tomatillo halves with nonstick cooking spray. Grill for 5 minutes, turning once. Cool slightly and cut into 1-inch pieces.

4 Place fish cubes on 4 metal skewers and grill for 5 minutes, turning once.

5 In bowl combine tomatillos, remaining 2 tablespoons cilantro, and 2 tablespoons green onion.

6 Lightly spray tortillas with nonstick cooking spray. Place tortillas on grill for 1 minute or until lightly toasted, turning once. Slide fish off skewers and serve in tortillas topped with salsa, sour cream, and avocado.

Makes 2 servings

COMPLETE MEAL SERVING
537 calories / 17 g total fat / 151 calories from fat / 26% calories from fat
172 mg cholesterol / 559 mg sodium / 60 g carbohydrate / 10 g fiber / 1 g sugars / 50 g protein

Seared Cod with Steamed Vegetables

Prep Time: 10 minutes ■ Cook Time: 11 minutes

Cooking meat, poultry, or fish quickly at a high temperature is known as searing, which creates a crust that seals in the natural juices. Searing results from roasting at high temperature, broiling, or, as in this recipe, cooking in a skillet over high heat, usually in a bit of oil.

¼	cup reduced-sodium soy sauce
¼	cup chopped green onion (2)
2	tablespoons chopped fresh ginger
1	teaspoon lime zest
2	tablespoons lime juice
2	teaspoons honey
	Nonstick cooking spray
4	6-ounce cod fillets
8	ounces snow peas, trimmed
1	carrot, sliced lengthwise and bias-sliced
3½	ounces shiitake mushrooms, stemmed and halved
½	cup chopped unsalted dry-roasted peanuts

1 In small bowl combine soy sauce, green onion, ginger, zest, lime juice, and honey; set aside.

2 In large skillet lightly sprayed with nonstick cooking spray cook cod over high heat for 6 minutes or until fish flakes easily when tested with fork, turning once; remove cod to serving plate; keep warm.

3 Add soy sauce mixture to skillet, scraping up any brown bits with wooden spoon. Add snow peas, carrot, and mushrooms; cover and cook vegetables for 5 minutes or until crisp-tender. Spoon vegetables and sauce over fish. Sprinkle with peanuts.

Makes 4 servings

to complete the meal   For 4 servings: 2 cups hot cooked quinoa

COMPLETE MEAL SERVING
432 calories / 12 g total fat / 110 calories from fat / 25% calories from fat
69 mg cholesterol / 737 mg sodium / 37 g carbohydrate / 6 g fiber / 6 g sugars / 45 g protein

Okra-Stuffed Trout

Prep Time: 10 minutes ■ Cook Time: 8 minutes

Baked trout fillets are delicious topped with a zesty okra-tomato mixture. Using frozen okra makes this meal ready in minutes.

	Nonstick cooking spray
4	6-ounce trout fillets
2	teaspoons garlic and herb seasoning blend
¼	teaspoon ground black pepper
2	cups frozen cut okra, thawed
2	cups chopped tomato
½	cup chopped onion (½ large)
6	cloves garlic, minced
2	tablespoons grated Parmesan cheese
1	teaspoon crushed red pepper flakes
1	teaspoon lemon zest
¼	teaspoon salt

1 Preheat oven to 400°F. Lightly spray large roasting pan with nonstick cooking spray.

2 Place trout in prepared pan. Rub both sides of trout with seasoning blend and black pepper.

3 In large bowl combine okra, tomato, onion, garlic, cheese, red pepper flakes, zest, and salt. Toss until well blended. Divide mixture over trout. Bake for 8 minutes or until vegetable mixture is hot and fish flakes easily when tested with fork.

Makes 4 servings

to complete the meal   For 4 servings: 1½ pounds cooked sweet potatoes, mashed and topped with ¼ cup chopped pecans

COMPLETE MEAL SERVING
422 calories / 15 g total fat / 131 calories from fat / 30% calories from fat
92 mg cholesterol / 287 mg sodium / 92 g carbohydrate / 8 g fiber / 16 g sugars / 36 g protein

Grouper with Strawberry-Mango Salsa

Prep Time: 10 minutes ■ Cook Time: 6 minutes

This cool salsa served on grilled fish is the perfect dinner for those hot summer nights when it feels too warm to cook. The strawberry-mango blend is a refreshing combination that pairs scrumptiously with chicken, pork, meat, and most kinds of fish.

Nonstick grilling spray

1 pound white fish such as Florida grouper, cut into 4 pieces

¼ teaspoon cracked black pepper

2 cups quartered strawberries

1 cup peeled, seeded, and chopped mango (1)

½ cup lime juice

½ teaspoon Vietnamese chili paste

1 tablespoon snipped fresh mint

1 tablespoon snipped fresh cilantro

½ cup chopped unsalted peanuts

1 Lightly spray grill grate with nonstick grilling spray and heat grill to medium.

2 Season fish with pepper.

3 In medium bowl combine strawberries, mango, lime juice, chili paste, mint, and cilantro. Set aside.

4 Grill fish for 6 minutes or until fish flakes easily when tested with fork, turning once.

5 Divide fish among 4 plates. Divide salsa onto each plate. Garnish with peanuts.

Makes 4 servings

to complete the meal For 4 servings: 2 cups hot cooked whole wheat couscous ■ 6 cups torn lettuce leaves tossed with ½ cup fat-free creamy Parmesan salad dressing and ½ cup grated low-fat Parmesan cheese

COMPLETE MEAL SERVING
515 calories / 15 g total fat / 131 calories from fat / 25% calories from fat
148 mg cholesterol / 575 mg sodium / 64 g carbohydrate / 11 g fiber / 17 g sugars / 37 g protein

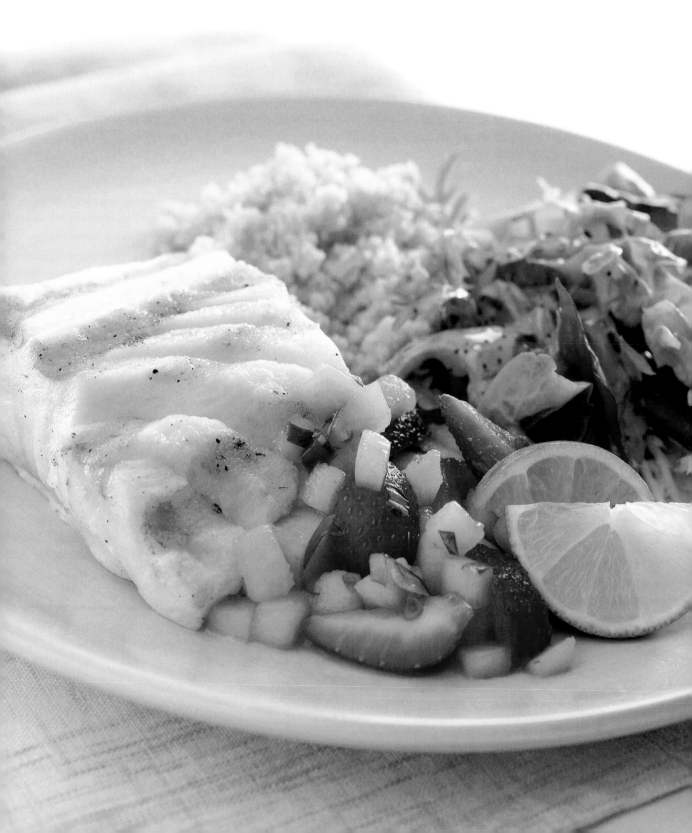

Fish with Citrus Sauce

Prep Time: 10 minutes ■ Cook Time: 10 minutes

Using freshly squeezed fruit juices for this marinade gives the dish a crisp flavor, but you can also use bottled juices. If you can't find tangerine juice, substitute orange or lemon juice or a combination of both.

½ cup tangerine juice

½ cup orange juice

3 tablespoons lime juice

2 tablespoons tequila

1 teaspoon ground cumin

1 teaspoon garlic powder

4 6-ounce fresh whitefish or halibut steaks

Nonstick grilling spray

1 In shallow glass baking dish whisk together tangerine juice, orange juice, lime juice, tequila, cumin, and garlic powder. Add fish; set aside to marinate for 15 minutes.

2 Lightly spray grill grate with nonstick grilling spray. Heat grill to medium.

3 Remove fish from marinade, reserving marinade. Grill fish for 7 minutes or until fish flakes easily when tested with fork, turning once.

4 Meanwhile, place reserved marinade in small saucepan; bring to boiling over high heat. Boil for 3 minutes or until slightly thickened. Serve over fish.

Makes 4 servings

to complete the meal   For 4 servings: 2 cups hot cooked brown rice ■ 1 small bunch broccoli, steamed and topped with 2 tablespoons slivered almonds

COMPLETE MEAL SERVING
418 calories / 13 g total fat / 120 calories from fat / 29% calories from fat
105 mg cholesterol / 114 mg sodium / 35 g carbohydrate / 5 g fiber / 8 g sugars / 39 g protein

Smoky Halibut Burgers

Prep Time: 5 minutes ■ Cook Time: 16 minutes

Chipotle peppers are dried smoked jalapeño peppers with dark, wrinkled skin. Their robust smoky flavor adds a wonderful richness to dishes. Just a little goes a long way when used as a seasoning.

	Nonstick cooking spray
1	1½-pound halibut fillet, cut into 4 equal pieces
⅓	cup low-fat mayonnaise
¼	cup chopped green onion (2)
1	tablespoon chipotle peppers in adobo sauce, finely chopped (see tip, page 34)
1	tablespoon lime juice
1	red onion, cut into ¼-inch slices
1	mango, peeled, seeded, and cut into ¼-inch slices
4	2-ounce onion rolls, halved
4	romaine lettuce leaves

1 Preheat broiler. Lightly spray rack of broiler pan with nonstick cooking spray.

2 Place fish on rack.

3 In small bowl combine mayonnaise, green onion, chipotle pepper in adobo sauce, and lime juice. Coat each piece of fish with one-fourth of the mayonnaise mixture.

4 Broil fish 5 inches from heat for 8 minutes or until fish flakes easily when tested with fork, turning once.

5 Meanwhile, in large nonstick skillet lightly sprayed with nonstick cooking spray cook red onion over medium-high heat for 5 minutes, turning once. Add mango and cook for 3 minutes or until brown and tender.

6 Fill rolls with lettuce, fish, mango, and onion.

Makes 4 servings

to complete the meal   For 4 servings: 4 cups coleslaw mix tossed with ¼ cup fat-free ranch salad dressing and 1 ounce grated reduced-fat cheddar cheese

COMPLETE MEAL SERVING
483 calories / 15 g total fat / 133 calories from fat / 28% calories from fat
62 mg cholesterol / 981 mg sodium / 47 g carbohydrate / 4 g fiber / 11 g sugars / 40 g protein

Seared Halibut with Lemon Sauce

Prep Time: 10 minutes ■ Cook Time: 10 minutes

The pickled buds of the caper plant, capers are a common seasoning in Mediterranean cooking, often adding a piquant flavor to sauces. Capers, available in several sizes, are packed in a salty brine sauce. Rinsing the capers before using them will remove some of the salt.

4	6-ounce halibut fillets, skinned
3	tablespoons seasoned bread crumbs
	Nonstick cooking spray
2	shallots, thinly sliced
1	clove garlic, minced
¼	cup chicken broth
¼	cup lemon juice
1	tablespoon honey
2	tablespoons drained capers
1	cup diced avocado

1 Evenly coat both sides of halibut fillets with bread crumbs.

2 In large nonstick skillet lightly sprayed with nonstick cooking spray cook halibut over medium-high heat for 8 minutes or until fish flakes easily when tested with fork, turning once. Remove halibut to serving plate and keep warm.

3 Lightly spray the same skillet with nonstick cooking spray. Add shallot and garlic; cook and stir for 1 minute. Add broth, lemon juice, honey, and capers. Bring to boiling; cook 1 minute. Pour over halibut. Garnish with avocado.

Makes 4 servings

to complete the meal For 4 servings: 8 ounces whole grain fusilli pasta, cooked ■ 8 ounces sugar snap peas, steamed and topped with ¼ cup slivered almonds

COMPLETE MEAL SERVING
582 calories / 16 g total fat / 147 calories from fat / 25% calories from fat
58 mg cholesterol / 566 mg sodium / 63 g carbohydrate / 16 g fiber / 10 g sugars / 50 g protein

Dilled Salmon Cakes

Prep Time: 10 minutes ■ Cook Time: 8 minutes

Canned salmon is available in three different types: pink, chum (keta), and red (sockeye). For soups, sandwiches, spreads, and patties, choose the pink or chum. Use red salmon for pastas, salads, or eating as is.

Sauce			*Cakes*		
	½	cup plain low-fat yogurt		2	14¾-ounce cans pink salmon, drained and skin and bones removed
	⅓	cup chopped, seeded tomato		¾	cup quick-cooking rolled oats
	⅓	cup chopped, seeded cucumber		⅓	cup low-fat (1%) milk
	1	tablespoon minced onion		2	egg whites
	1	tablespoon snipped fresh dill or 1 teaspoon dried dillweed, crushed		2	tablespoons finely chopped onion
				1	tablespoon snipped fresh dill or 1 teaspoon dried dillweed, crushed Nonstick cooking spray

1 To make the sauce, in small bowl stir together yogurt, tomato, cucumber, onion, and dill. Cover and refrigerate.

2 To make the cakes, in medium bowl combine salmon, oats, milk, egg whites, onion, and dill; mix well. Let stand for 5 minutes. Shape into five 1-inch-thick oval cakes.

3 In large skillet lightly sprayed with nonstick cooking spray cook salmon cakes over medium heat for 8 minutes or until golden brown and heated through, turning once. Place on 5 plates and divide sauce onto cakes.

Makes 5 servings

to complete the meal   For 5 servings: 5 ounces French bread ■ 5 cups salad greens tossed with ½ cup creamy fat-free Italian dressing and ¼ cup chopped pecans

COMPLETE MEAL SERVING
398 calories / 12 g total fat / 105 calories from fat / 26% calories from fat
99 mg cholesterol / 1,008 mg sodium / 32 g carbohydrate / 4 g fiber / 5 g sugars / 43 g protein

Barbecued Salmon with Collards, Okra, and Tomato

Prep Time: 15 minutes ■ Cook Time: 15 minutes

Be sure to buy wild salmon because it's leaner than farm-raised. Wild salmon is available fresh from May to October, so you may opt for frozen wild salmon that's available year-round.

    4 6-ounce wild salmon fillets
    ¼ cup smoky barbecue sauce
       Nonstick cooking spray
    1 pound collard greens, shredded
    1 10-ounce box frozen cut okra
    2 cups chopped tomato (3 medium)

1 Preheat broiler. Place salmon on rack of broiler pan and brush with barbecue sauce. Broil 4 inches from heat for 5 minutes or until fish flakes easily when tested with fork.

2 Meanwhile, in large skillet lightly sprayed with nonstick cooking spray cook collard greens over medium-high heat, turning frequently with tongs for 5 minutes or until wilted. Add okra and tomato; cook and stir for 5 minutes or until collard greens are tender.

Makes 4 servings

to complete the meal For 4 servings: 2 cups hot cooked quick-cooking brown rice tossed with ¼ cup chopped pecans

COMPLETE MEAL SERVING
386 calories / 13 g total fat / 114 calories from fat / 29% calories from fat
80 mg cholesterol / 319 mg sodium / 30 g carbohydrate / 7 g fiber / 8 g sugars / 40 g protein

moving forward
Eat without engaging in other activities: no reading, watching television, or Internet surfing.

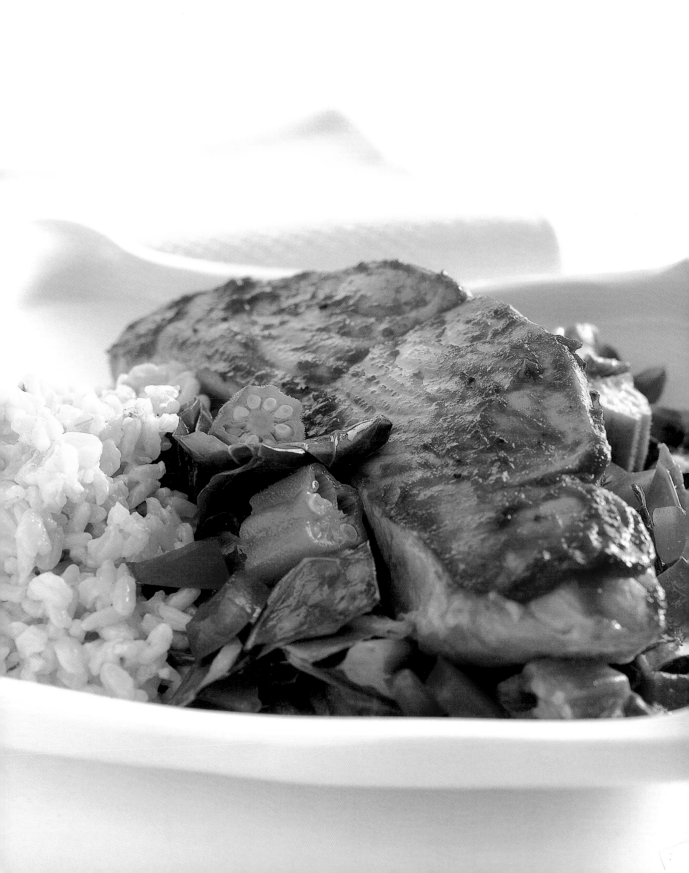

Baked Salmon with Asparagus and Sweet Potatoes

Prep Time: 10 minutes ■ Cook Time: 12 minutes

Preparing this meal amounts to seasoning a piece of fish, peeling and slicing a sweet potato, and washing some asparagus. For that minimum effort, you get maximum results!

	Nonstick cooking spray
1	1½-pound wild salmon fillet, cut into 4 equal pieces
¼	teaspoon salt
½	teaspoon ground black pepper
1	pound asparagus, trimmed
1	large sweet potato (1 pound), peeled and cut into ¼-inch slices
2	tablespoons sesame seeds

1 Preheat oven to 450°F. Lightly spray jelly-roll pan with nonstick cooking spray.

2 Place salmon, skin sides down, on one side of prepared pan and season with ⅛ teaspoon of the salt and one-third of the pepper.

3 Place asparagus in single layer on other side of pan and sprinkle with one-third of the pepper. Gently toss asparagus to coat.

4 Lightly spray a second jelly-roll pan with nonstick cooking spray. Place potato on pan and sprinkle with remaining ⅛ teaspoon salt and remaining pepper.

5 Place both pans in oven and roast for 12 to 15 minutes, turning the asparagus and potato once, until fish flakes easily when tested with fork. Garnish with sesame seeds.

Makes 4 servings

to complete the meal   Per serving: one 1-ounce whole wheat roll spread with
½ teaspoon trans-fat-free canola margarine

COMPLETE MEAL SERVING
403 calories / 12 g total fat / 109 calories from fat / 27% calories from fat
80 mg cholesterol / 356 mg sodium / 33 g carbohydrate / 12 g fiber / 10 g sugars / 40 g protein

Corn Cakes with Salmon and Dill

Prep Time: 15 minutes ■ Cook Time: 9 minutes

Here's a great way to use up leftover salmon. Be sure to grill or broil extra salmon next time and then save 4 ounces for this quick, delicious meal later in the week.

1 cup yellow cornmeal
⅓ cup all-purpose flour
2 tablespoons sugar
1 teaspoon baking powder
1 cup low-fat (1%) milk
½ cup egg substitute
⅓ cup chopped green onion (3)
   Nonstick cooking spray
¾ cup reduced-fat sour cream
1 4-ounce cooked salmon fillet
   Fresh snipped dill

1 In large bowl combine cornmeal, flour, sugar, and baking powder until blended.

2 In medium bowl whisk together milk and egg substitute; stir in green onion. Stir milk mixture into flour mixture just until blended.

3 Preheat oven to 200°F. Lightly spray large nonstick skillet with nonstick cooking spray and place over medium heat until hot. For each corn cake, spoon about 2 tablespoons batter into skillet. Cook for 2 minutes or until bubbles appear on top and the edges are barely dry. Turn; cook for 1 minute or until the center springs back when touched. Place on ovenproof plate and keep warm in oven. Repeat with remaining batter, lightly spraying skillet with nonstick cooking spray as needed.

4 To serve, place 3 cakes on each of 4 plates. Top each cake with 1 tablespoon sour cream and place one-fourth of the salmon on each plate. Serve with dill.

Makes 4 servings

to complete the meal For 4 servings: 4 cups salad greens and 1 chopped tomato tossed with ¼ cup fat-free balsamic vinaigrette and ¼ cup sliced almonds

COMPLETE MEAL SERVING
412 calories / 12 g total fat / 106 calories from fat / 26% calories from fat
39 mg cholesterol / 399 mg sodium / 57 g carbohydrate / 5 g fiber / 15 g sugars / 21 g protein

Seared Scallops over Chard

Prep Time: 10 minutes ■ Cook Time: 13 minutes

There are two types of scallops: bay and sea scallops. Bay (or calico) scallops, typically found only on the East Coast, are very small and sweeter and juicier than sea scallops. Much larger, sea scallops have a sweet, tender meat with a chewier texture than the bay variety.

1½	pounds Swiss chard, stem ends trimmed
	Nonstick cooking spray
1	cup chopped red sweet pepper (1)
1	clove garlic, pressed
¼	cup chopped dried apricots
⅓	cup pine nuts, toasted
1¼	pounds sea scallops, side hinges removed

1 Remove stems from chard and coarsely chop leaves and stems.

2 In medium saucepan cook chard and stems over high heat in enough boiling water to cover for 10 minutes; drain well.

3 Meanwhile, in large skillet lightly sprayed with nonstick cooking spray cook and stir sweet pepper and garlic over medium-high heat for 3 minutes or until light brown. Add chard; cook and stir for 3 minutes or until vegetables are tender. Stir in apricots and pine nuts.

4 While chard is cooking, pat scallops dry with paper towels.

5 In large skillet lightly sprayed with nonstick cooking spray cook scallops in batches over medium-high heat for 3 minutes or until opaque, turning once.

6 Divide chard mixture onto 4 plates. Divide scallops and any juices that have accumulated over chard.

Makes 4 servings

to complete the meal   For 4 servings: 2 cups hot cooked whole wheat couscous tossed with ¼ cup raisins and ¼ cup sliced almonds

COMPLETE MEAL SERVING
478 calories / 14 g total fat / 128 calories from fat / 26% calories from fat
46 mg cholesterol / 545 mg sodium / 57 g carbohydrate / 11 g fiber / 13 g sugars / 36 g protein

Steamed Sea Bass with Creamy Buttermilk Coleslaw

Prep Time: 10 minutes ■ Cook Time: 2 minutes

Sea bass, often hailing from Chile, has a moderately firm texture and mild flavor. If you can't find it, substitute swordfish, halibut, or salmon.

¼	cup low-fat buttermilk
½	cup low-fat sour cream
1½	tablespoons Dijon honey mustard
½	16-ounce package coleslaw mix
½	cup dried cranberries
⅓	cup slivered almonds
4	5-ounce fresh or frozen sea bass fillets
¼	teaspoon ground black pepper

1 In large bowl whisk together buttermilk, sour cream, and honey mustard. Add coleslaw mix, cranberries, and almonds. Toss to coat well. Refrigerate until ready to serve.

2 Place bass on large microwave-safe plate with the thickest parts at the edge of the plate. Season with pepper. Cover with microwave-safe plastic wrap. Microwave on 100% power (high) for 2 to 4 minutes or until fish flakes easily when tested with fork.

Makes 4 servings

to complete the meal   For 4 servings: 2 cups hot cooked whole wheat noodles

COMPLETE MEAL SERVING
440 calories / 13 g total fat / 117 calories from fat / 26% calories from fat
72 mg cholesterol / 190 mg sodium / 46 g carbohydrate / 6 g fiber / 20 g sugars / 36 g protein

moving forward

When you get the munchies, distract yourself with an activity you enjoy. Take a walk, do some gardening, or go for a bike ride.

Linguine with Shrimp Scampi

Prep Time: 3 minutes ■ Cook Time: 10 minutes

Keep a bag of peeled and deveined uncooked shrimp in your freezer for last-minute dinners. Whole grain pastas have more fiber and nutrients than regular, so switch your family to this variety. It may help to start by using half whole grain and half regular, eventually switching to all whole grain.

8	ounces whole grain linguine
	Nonstick cooking spray
¾	pound peeled and deveined large shrimp
¼	teaspoon ground black pepper
2	tablespoons chopped garlic
⅔	cup dry white wine
2	tablespoons snipped fresh flat-leaf parsley
1½	teaspoons snipped fresh thyme
1	teaspoon grated lemon zest
½	cup grated Parmesan cheese

1 Prepare pasta according to package directions. Drain, reserving 1 cup pasta water. Return pasta to pot.

2 Meanwhile, in large skillet lightly sprayed with nonstick cooking spray cook shrimp over medium-high heat for 3 minutes or until shrimp are opaque. With slotted spoon, remove shrimp to bowl.

3 Add pepper and garlic and cook for 1 minute. Add wine, parsley, thyme, and zest; heat to boiling over high heat. Cook for 1 minute, stirring occasionally.

4 Return shrimp to skillet; cook for 1 minute to heat through. Pour over linguine in pot, adding half of the reserved pasta water. Toss to coat; add more pasta water if needed. Sprinkle with cheese.

Makes 4 servings

to complete the meal   For 4 servings: 6 cups torn mixed salad greens tossed with ⅓ cup fat-free Caesar dressing and ½ cup pine nuts

COMPLETE MEAL SERVING
428 calories / 14 g total fat / 122 calories from fat / 27% calories from fat
134 mg cholesterol / 672 mg sodium / 52 g carbohydrate / 9 g fiber / 5 g sugars / 30 g protein

Gazpacho with Spicy Shrimp

Prep Time: 10 minutes ■ Cook Time: 2 minutes

This flavorful Spanish-inspired dinner is perfect for hot summer nights when heating up the kitchen isn't an option. Just light up the grill while you blend gazpacho ingredients and you'll have a light, refreshing meal in less than 15 minutes!

1	pound peeled and deveined extra-large shrimp
2	teaspoons hot pepper sauce
¾	cup chopped green onion (6)
7	tablespoons snipped fresh cilantro
3	cups chopped English cucumber (2)
6	medium tomatillos (1 pound), chopped
2	tablespoons white wine vinegar
2	teaspoons sugar
	Nonstick grilling spray
½	cup sour cream
½	cup diced avocado

1 In small bowl combine shrimp, pepper sauce, 1 tablespoon of the green onion, and 1 tablespoon of the cilantro; set aside.

2 Meanwhile, in food processor process cucumber, tomatillo, vinegar, sugar, remaining green onion, and remaining cilantro until smooth.

3 Lightly spray grill grate with nonstick grilling spray and heat to medium-high. Grill shrimp for 2 minutes, turning once. Coarsely chop shrimp.

4 Ladle gazpacho into serving bowls. Top each with 2 tablespoons sour cream. Divide grilled shrimp and avocado among bowls.

Makes 4 servings

to complete the meal Per serving: one 2-ounce seven-grain roll

COMPLETE MEAL SERVING
386 calories / 13 g total fat / 119 calories from fat / 30% calories from fat
181 mg cholesterol / 554 mg sodium / 43 g carbohydrate / 8 g fiber / 8 g sugars / 28 g protein

Citrus Shrimp and Couscous Toss

Prep Time: 20 minutes ■ Cook Time: 10 minutes

Couscous is pasta made from tiny granules of semolina. It's a staple in many cuisines around the world. It has a light, fluffy texture and often takes the place of rice, potatoes, or other types of pasta.

2	large oranges
1	large red grapefruit
1	pound peeled and deveined large shrimp
½	cup uncooked whole wheat couscous
2	cups chopped fennel (2)
¼	cup chopped red onion
½	cup chopped, pitted kalamata olives
½	cup slivered almonds
	Nonstick cooking spray
⅓	cup fat-free balsamic vinaigrette
½	large head Boston lettuce, separated into leaves

1 Grate enough zest from 1 orange to measure 2½ teaspoons. Remove peel and pith from oranges and grapefruit. Working over a bowl to catch any juices, cut oranges and grapefruit into segments. Squeeze the orange and grapefruit membranes to extract any remaining juice.

2 Place shrimp in resealable plastic bag. Add 2 tablespoons orange and grapefruit juice mixture and 1 teaspoon zest.

3 Prepare couscous according to package directions, replacing 6 tablespoons of water with 6 tablespoons of orange and grapefruit juice mixture. Place couscous in large bowl with fennel, onion, olives, and almonds.

4 In large nonstick skillet lightly sprayed with nonstick cooking spray cook and stir shrimp over medium-high heat for 5 minutes or until opaque. Add shrimp to bowl with couscous.

5 In small bowl stir remaining 1½ teaspoons zest into dressing. Pour dressing over couscous mixture. Toss to coat.

6 Evenly divide lettuce among four plates. Divide couscous mixture on top of each plate.

Makes 4 servings

to complete the meal   Per serving: two 7⅝×⅝-inch breadsticks

COMPLETE MEAL SERVING
518 calories / 15 g total fat / 136 calories from fat / 25% calories from fat
168 mg cholesterol / 823 mg sodium / 70 g carbohydrate / 11 g fiber / 21 g sugars / 30 g protein

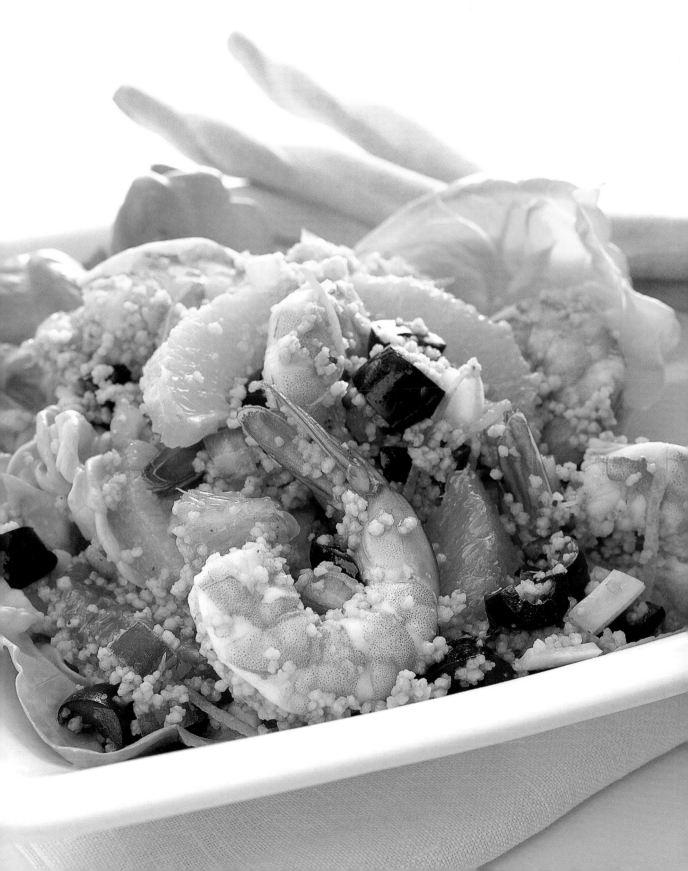

Pan-Roasted Tuna with Grapefruit and Leeks

Prep Time: 15 minutes ■ Cook Time: 13 minutes

Available whole and ground, fennel seeds add a mild anise flavor to both sweet and savory dishes. To crush the seeds, use a mortar and pestle or place them in a resealable plastic bag and very firmly press a heavy skillet onto the seeds, twisting as you press.

1	teaspoon fennel seeds, crushed
¼	teaspoon ground black pepper
4	6-ounce tuna steaks
	Nonstick cooking spray
2	leeks, green ends discarded and white ends halved, rinsed, and thinly sliced (1 cup)
1	tablespoon chopped fresh ginger
1	teaspoon finely chopped jalapeño pepper (see tip, page 34)
1	teaspoon olive oil
1	medium grapefruit, sectioned and then sections halved (about 1 cup sections)
1	teaspoon sugar

1 In small bowl combine fennel seeds and black pepper. Rub onto sides of tuna.

2 In large nonstick skillet lightly sprayed with nonstick cooking spray cook tuna over medium-high heat for 10 minutes or until fish flakes easily when tested with fork, turning once. Remove tuna to serving plate; keep warm.

3 In same skillet cook and stir leek, ginger, and jalapeño over medium heat in hot oil for 3 minutes. Remove from heat and stir in grapefruit and sugar. Pour over tuna.

Makes 4 servings

to complete the meal For 4 servings: 1 pound frozen steak fries, baked ■ 1 pound green beans, steamed

COMPLETE MEAL SERVING
482 calories / 14 g total fat / 123 calories from fat / 26% calories from fat
63 mg cholesterol / 99 mg sodium / 46 g carbohydrate / 10 g fiber / 9 g sugars / 44 g protein

Pan-Fried Catfish

Prep Time: 5 minutes ■ Cook Time: 11 minutes

Here's a healthy take on deep-fried Southern catfish that your whole family will love. Try to use fresh lemon juice because it makes a superior sauce than bottled lemon juice. Go for fresh limes if you're out of lemons.

        Nonstick cooking spray
½   cup yellow cornmeal
2   teaspoons paprika
¼   teaspoon ground black pepper
⅛   teaspoon cayenne pepper
½   cup fat-free (skim) milk
1   pound wild catfish, flounder, cod, or orange roughy fillets
½   cup lemon juice
2   tablespoons snipped fresh Italian parsley
2   tablespoons snipped fresh chives
2   teaspoons capers, drained

1 Preheat oven to 300°F. Lightly spray 2 baking sheets with nonstick cooking spray.

2 In large resealable plastic bag combine cornmeal, paprika, black pepper, and cayenne pepper.

3 Place milk in shallow dish. Working with one fillet at a time, dip fish into milk until coated. Place in bag with cornmeal, gently turning until well coated. Place on first baking sheet. Repeat with remaining fish fillets and cornmeal mixture.

4 Heat large nonstick skillet lightly sprayed with nonstick cooking spray over medium-high heat. Place 2 fillets in skillet; lightly spray fillets with nonstick cooking spray. Cook for 5 minutes or until golden and fish flakes easily when tested with fork, turning once. Remove to second baking sheet. Place in oven to keep warm. Repeat with remaining fish.

5 Increase heat to high. Add lemon juice, parsley, chives, and capers to skillet. Cook and stir for 1 minute or until slightly thickened. Place fish on serving plate and drizzle with sauce.

Makes 4 servings

to complete the meal   For 4 servings: 12 ounces frozen tater tots, cooked ■ one 16-ounce bag frozen broccoli, corn, and sweet peppers, cooked

COMPLETE MEAL SERVING
393 calories / 13 g total fat / 113 calories from fat / 29% calories from fat
66 mg cholesterol / 473 mg sodium / 52 g carbohydrate / 7 g fiber / 6 g sugars / 26 g protein

Spring Vegetable Lasagna

Prep Time: 10 minutes ■ Cook Time: 35 minutes

Vegetables layered with rich ricotta and Parmesan cheeses and noodles, then bathed in marinara sauce make a delicious, satisfying meal that's sure to please the whole family.

	Nonstick cooking spray
3	1-pound bags Italian blend frozen vegetables
1	tablespoon dried thyme, crushed
1½	15-ounce containers part-skim ricotta cheese
1	cup grated Parmesan cheese
1	egg
4	cups low-sodium, low-fat marinara sauce
1	8-ounce box oven-ready lasagna noodles
2	cups part-skim shredded mozzarella

1 Preheat oven to 350°F. Lightly spray 13×9-inch baking dish with nonstick cooking spray.

2 In large skillet lightly sprayed with nonstick cooking spray cook vegetables and 2 teaspoons of the thyme over high heat for 5 minutes or until vegetables are crisp-tender.

3 In medium bowl combine ricotta cheese, Parmesan cheese, egg, and the remaining 1 teaspoon thyme.

4 Spread ½ cup marinara sauce on bottom of prepared pan. Place 3 uncooked noodles crosswise over sauce. Spread 1 cup ricotta mixture over pasta. Top with one-third (about 2 cups) vegetables. Sprinkle ⅔ cup mozzarella evenly over vegetables. Spread 1 cup marinara sauce over vegetables and mozzarella. Repeat layers twice. Top with the remaining 3 pasta pieces and remaining ½ cup marinara sauce. Cover with foil and bake for 30 minutes or until hot and bubbly. Let stand 10 minutes before cutting.

Makes 12 servings

to complete the meal   Per serving: 1 slice French bread

COMPLETE MEAL SERVING
371 calories / 12 g total fat / 105 calories from fat / 29% calories from fat
50 mg cholesterol / 564 mg sodium / 44 g carbohydrate / 5 g fiber / 9 g sugars / 21 g protein

Buffalo Macaroni and Cheese

Prep Time: 5 minutes ■ Cook Time: 11 minutes

If you love the flavors of buffalo chicken wings, here's a creamy baked macaroni dish reminiscent of these rich flavors. Your family will love the tastes of the cheeses and hot pepper sauce blended with penne pasta.

- 1 13¼-ounce box whole wheat blend penne pasta
- 2 tablespoons all-purpose flour
- ¼ teaspoon ground black pepper
- 2 cups reduced-fat (2%) milk
- ¼ cup reduced-calorie tub-style cream cheese (Neufchâtel)
- 4 ounces shredded low-fat, reduced-sodium cheddar cheese
- 4 ounces low-fat goat cheese
- 2 tablespoons buffalo wing sauce

1 Cook pasta according to package directions.

2 Meanwhile, place flour and pepper in large saucepan. Add milk, stirring with a whisk until blended. Drop cream cheese by tablespoonfuls into milk mixture; bring to boiling over medium-high heat, stirring constantly. Reduce heat; simmer 2 minutes or until thick and cream cheese melts, stirring occasionally.

3 Remove from heat and stir in cheddar cheese, goat cheese, wing sauce, and pasta.

Makes 4 servings

to complete the meal For 4 servings: 6 cups mixed salad greens tossed with ⅓ cup fat-free ranch dressing and ¼ cup chopped walnuts

COMPLETE MEAL SERVING
598 calories / 17 g total fat / 158 calories from fat / 25% calories from fat
32 mg cholesterol / 706 mg sodium / 93 g carbohydrate / 13 g fiber / 11 g sugars / 27 g protein

moving forward
Watch what you eat…literally. Plate your food instead of eating it out of a bag.

Fettuccine with Asparagus

Prep Time: 5 minutes ▪ Cook Time: 11 minutes

Many recipes call for the addition of citrus zest, most often lemon or orange, because it adds great fresh flavor. However, if you don't have fresh fruits and are using bottled juice instead, you can eliminate the zest and still enjoy a great-tasting meal.

12	ounces uncooked fettuccine pasta
1	pound asparagus, trimmed and cut into 1-inch pieces
1	orange sweet pepper, cut into ¼-inch slices
1	tablespoon trans-fat-free canola margarine
1	tablespoon all-purpose flour
¼	teaspoon ground black pepper
2	cups evaporated low-fat (1%) milk
1	6½-ounce box light garlic and herbs low-fat spreadable cheese
4	ounces baked smoked tofu
2	tablespoons snipped fresh dill
1	tablespoon lemon juice
1	teaspoon lemon zest
¼	cup pine nuts
6	tablespoons grated Parmesan cheese

1 Prepare pasta according to package directions, adding asparagus and sweet pepper to pasta during last 3 minutes of pasta cooking time. Drain; place in large serving bowl.

2 Meanwhile, melt margarine in large saucepan. Whisk in flour and black pepper until well blended. Cook for 1 minute. Whisk in milk, stirring until blended. Bring to boiling over medium-high heat, stirring constantly. Remove from heat and add spreadable cheese 1 tablespoon at a time, stirring after each addition until smooth. Add tofu, dill, lemon juice, and zest. Cook for 1 minute to heat through. Pour over pasta and toss to coat well. Garnish with pine nuts and sprinkle with Parmesan cheese.

Makes 6 servings

COMPLETE MEAL SERVING
439 calories / 13 g total fat / 117 calories from fat / 26% calories from fat
23 mg cholesterol / 434 mg sodium / 57 g carbohydrate / 3 g fiber / 12 g sugars / 25 g protein

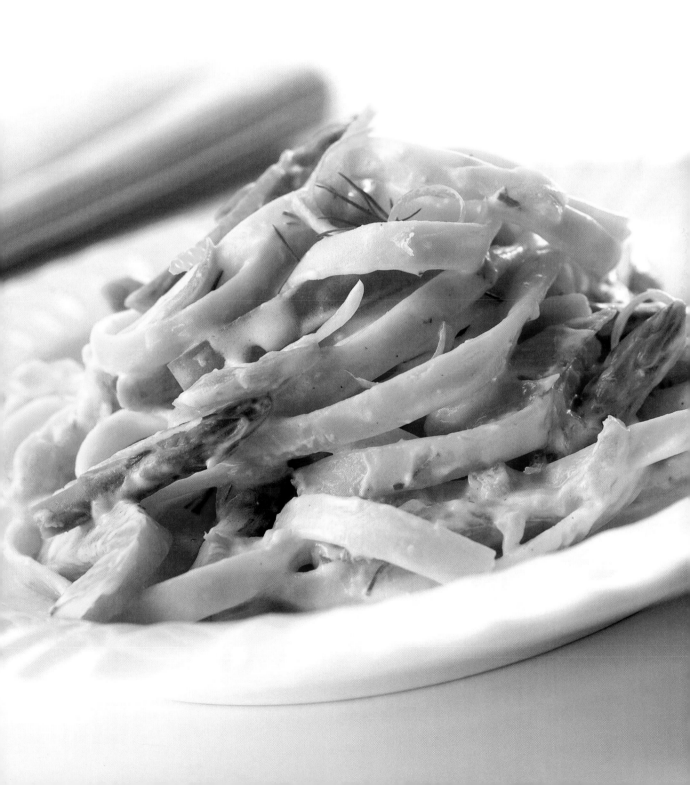

Farfalle Primavera

Prep Time: 20 minutes ■ Cook Time: 10 minutes

A simple way to trim asparagus is to tightly hold the spear end with one hand and the tough bottom with the other hand. Gently snap the spear; it will break, easily separating the tender portion from the tough end, which should be discarded.

8	ounces uncooked farfalle pasta
¾	pound trimmed asparagus spears, cut into 1-inch pieces
1	cup frozen peas
¼	cup fat-free vinaigrette
3	tomatoes, cut into ½-inch pieces
½	cup fresh basil leaves, torn
½	cup grated Parmesan cheese
½	cup pine nuts

1 Prepare pasta according to package directions, adding the asparagus and peas during the last 5 minutes of pasta cooking time. Drain.

2 Meanwhile, in large bowl pour vinaigrette. Add pasta mixture, tomato, and basil. Toss well and sprinkle with cheese and pine nuts.

Makes 4 servings

COMPLETE MEAL SERVING
431 calories / 13 g total fat / 117 calories from fat / 27% calories from fat
8 mg cholesterol / 358 mg sodium / 61 g carbohydrate / 6 g fiber / 11 g sugars / 20 g protein

moving forward

If you realize that you're overeating during stressful times, find another outlet to relax. Go for a walk, talk to friends, or write in a journal.

Orecchiette with Leeks and Edamame

Prep Time: 8 minutes ■ Cook Time: 15 minutes

Orecchiette pasta, "little ears" in Italian, is often prepared with thick, chunky sauces or in salads. Here it is tossed with edamame, leeks, and lemon for a flavorful meal.

8	ounces uncooked orecchiette pasta
1½	cups frozen edamame
1½	pounds leeks, well rinsed and chopped
1	teaspoon olive oil
2	tablespoons reduced-sodium vegetable broth
2	tablespoons lemon juice
1	tablespoon lemon zest
¼	teaspoon ground black pepper
¾	cup grated Parmesan cheese

1 Prepare pasta according to package directions, adding edamame during last 5 minutes of pasta cooking time. Drain, reserving ½ cup of the cooking water.

2 Meanwhile, in large nonstick skillet cook and stir leek in hot oil over medium-high heat for 3 minutes. Add broth; cover and cook for 8 minutes or until leek is tender.

3 Add pasta and edamame to skillet with ¼ cup of the reserved water. Stir in lemon juice, zest, and pepper. Cook for 3 minutes or until heated through, adding remaining ¼ cup pasta water if needed. Remove from heat and stir in cheese.

Makes 6 servings

to complete the meal For 6 servings: 6 slices whole grain bread ■ 6 cups salad greens tossed with ½ cup fat-free balsamic vinaigrette, ½ cup sliced almonds, and ½ cup sliced black olives

COMPLETE MEAL SERVING
425 calories / 12 g total fat / 111 calories from fat / 26% calories from fat
8 mg cholesterol / 660 mg sodium / 62 g carbohydrate / 8 g fiber / 11 g sugars / 19 g protein

Eggplant Curry

Prep Time: 10 minutes ■ Cook Time: 15 minutes

Garbanzo beans, also called chickpeas, are round tan beans with a nutty flavor and firm texture. They are common in Mediterranean, Indian, and Middle Eastern cuisines and make a delicious addition to soups, salads, and stews.

	Nonstick cooking spray
1	medium eggplant (8 ounces), peeled and cut into 1-inch pieces
1	cup bias-sliced carrot (2)
1	cup chopped onion (1 large)
1	teaspoon olive oil
1	tablespoon curry powder
1	tablespoon all-purpose flour
1	cup vegetable broth
1	cup reduced-fat (2%) milk
1	19-ounce can garbanzo beans, rinsed and drained
¼	cup snipped fresh cilantro

1 Preheat oven to 375°F. Lightly spray jelly-roll pan with nonstick cooking spray.

2 Place eggplant on prepared pan and lightly spray with nonstick cooking spray. Bake for 10 minutes or until tender.

3 Meanwhile, in large skillet cook and stir carrot and onion in hot oil over medium heat for 5 minutes or until brown. Add curry powder and flour; cook 1 minute. Whisk in broth and milk. Bring to boiling over high heat. Cook for 2 minutes, stirring constantly.

4 Add eggplant and beans. Reduce heat to low; cover and simmer for 5 minutes or until flavors blend. Stir in cilantro.

Makes 2 servings

to complete the meal For 2 servings: 4 cups chopped romaine lettuce with 3 tablespoons Italian dressing and 2 tablespoons pine nuts

COMPLETE MEAL SERVING
447 calories / 13 g total fat / 116 calories from fat / 25% calories from fat
11 mg cholesterol / 985 mg sodium / 66 g carbohydrate / 17 g fiber / 25 g sugars / 21 g protein

Teriyaki Tofu and Broccoli

Prep Time: 10 minutes ■ Cook Time: 10 minutes

Baked tofu is seasoned cooked tofu. It has a firm texture and mild flavor. Available in a variety of flavors and ready to eat, it's delicious on salads or tossed into soups or stir-fries.

　　　Nonstick cooking spray
1　8-ounce package teriyaki-flavored baked tofu, cut into 1-inch pieces
1　pound broccoli, cut into florets
2　large carrots, peeled and sliced
1　teaspoon olive oil
¼　cup reduced-sodium vegetable broth
1　tablespoon stir-fry sauce
2　cups cooked brown rice

1 In large nonstick wok or skillet lightly sprayed with nonstick cooking spray cook tofu over medium-high heat for 2 minutes or until heated through, stirring constantly. Remove to plate.

2 In same skillet or wok cook broccoli and carrot in hot oil for 2 minutes, stirring constantly. Add broth and stir-fry sauce. Cover and cook for 5 minutes or until vegetables are tender. Return tofu to skillet; cook for 1 minute to heat through.

3 Divide rice between 2 plates. Divide tofu mixture over rice.

Makes 2 servings

COMPLETE MEAL SERVING
524 calories / 15 g total fat / 136 calories from fat / 25% calories from fat
0 mg cholesterol / 902 mg sodium / 70 g carbohydrate / 14 g fiber / 10 g sugars / 31 g protein

moving forward
Don't be discouraged by little slips. There may be bumps in the road, but you can still keep moving forward.

Tomato and White Bean Chowder

Prep Time: 8 minutes ■ Cook Time: 15 minutes

Cannellini beans are white kidney beans used most often in soups and salads. The canned beans are quite tender and great for this soup, but you could substitute kidney or white beans, if desired.

1 cup chopped onion (1 large)
1 medium zucchini, halved lengthwise and cut into ¼-inch slices (1½ cups)
2 cloves garlic, chopped
1 teapoon olive oil
2 14½-ounce cans no-salt-added chopped tomatoes, undrained
2 16-ounce cans no-salt-added cannellini beans, rinsed and drained
2 cups reduced-sodium vegetable broth
2 tablespoons snipped fresh basil
¾ teaspoon Italian seasoning
6 tablespoons grated Parmesan cheese

1 In large saucepan cook and stir onion, zucchini, and garlic in hot oil over medium heat for 5 minutes or until tender. Add tomatoes, beans, broth, basil, and Italian seasoning; bring to boiling. Reduce heat to low and simmer for 10 minutes.

2 Divide among 6 bowls and top each bowl with 1 tablespoon cheese.

Makes 6 servings

to complete the meal For 6 servings: one 5-ounce package baby spinach tossed with ½ red onion, sliced; ½ cup jarred mandarin orange sections, drained; 2 hard-cooked eggs, sliced; and 1½ cups sliced avocado and drizzled with ¼ cup fat-free French dressing ■ six 2-ounce slices whole grain bread spread with 3 teaspoons trans-fat-free canola margarine

COMPLETE MEAL SERVING
482 calories / 14 g total fat / 128 calories from fat / 26% calories from fat
75 mg cholesterol / 737 mg sodium / 71 g carbohydrate / 16 g fiber / 19 g sugars / 22 g protein

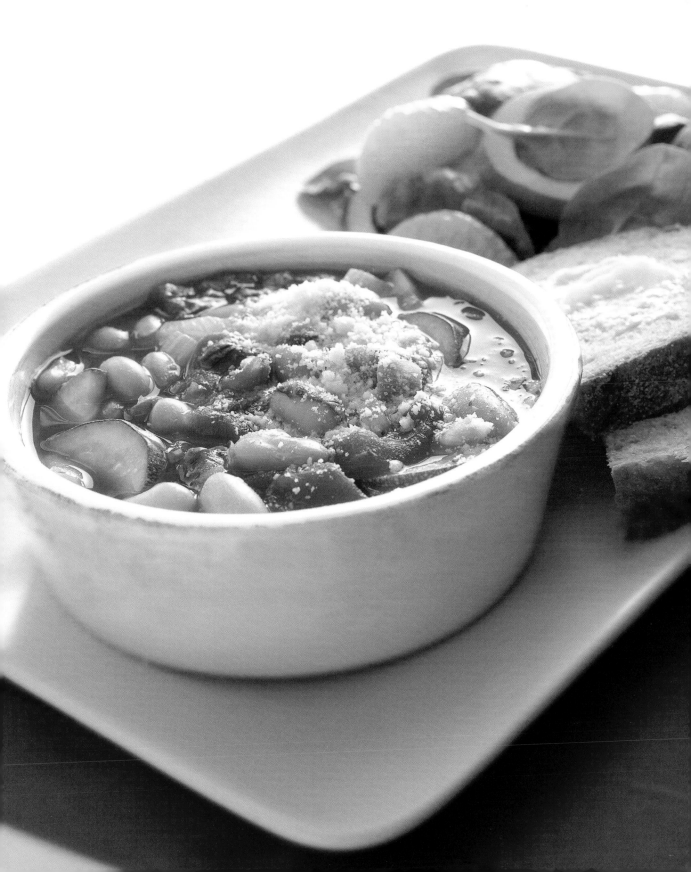

Broccoli Rabe, Garbanzo, and Penne

Prep Time: 10 minutes ■ Cook Time: 20 minutes

Broccoli rabe, also called raab or rapini, is a leafy green vegetable often used in Italian cooking. It has a pungent bitter taste and is often steamed or sauteed in olive oil and then tossed with pasta, garlic, and olive oil.

1	pound broccoli rabe, trimmed, washed, and cut into 1-inch pieces
8	ounces uncooked penne pasta
3	cloves garlic, thinly sliced
1	teaspoon olive oil
1	19-ounce can garbanzo beans, rinsed and drained
½	cup low-sodium vegetable broth
¼	teaspoon crushed red pepper flakes
½	cup grated Parmesan cheese
½	cup sliced black olives
⅓	cup pine nuts

1 Cook broccoli rabe in large saucepan with enough boiling water to cover for 5 minutes or until just crisp. Drain and set aside.

2 In same pan prepare pasta according to package directions. Drain; place in large serving bowl.

3 Meanwhile, in large skillet cook and stir garlic in hot oil over medium heat for 1 minute or until golden. Add beans, broth, and red pepper flakes. Simmer for 5 minutes, stirring occasionally. Add broccoli rabe and cook for 3 minutes or until tender. Pour over pasta and top with cheese, olives, and pine nuts. Toss to coat well.

Makes 4 servings

COMPLETE MEAL SERVING
466 calories / 14 g total fat / 123 calories from fat / 26% calories from fat
8 mg cholesterol / 705 mg sodium / 65 g carbohydrate / 7 g fiber / 6 g sugars / 23 g protein

Quick Lentil Stew

Prep Time: 10 minutes ■ Cook Time: 20 minutes

Look for ready-to-serve brown rice on supermarket shelves with the other rice products. It doesn't need refrigeration prior to opening and allows you to have brown rice available whenever you need it.

- 1   cup chopped onion (1 large)
- 1   clove garlic, minced
- 1   large carrot, cut into ½-inch slices
- 1   teaspoon olive oil
- 1   cup low-fat evaporated milk
- 2   15-ounce cans lentils
- 1   14½-ounce can no-salt-added diced tomatoes, undrained
- 2   4.4-ounce containers ready-to-serve brown rice

1 In Dutch oven or large saucepan cook onion, garlic, and carrot in hot oil over medium-high heat for 5 minutes, stirring frequently.

2 Stir in milk, lentils, and tomatoes. Bring to boiling over medium-high heat. Reduce heat to low; cover and simmer for 15 minutes to blend flavors.

3 Divide rice among 4 bowls. Divide stew over rice.

Makes 4 servings

to complete the meal For 4 servings: 6 cups mesclun tossed with ⅓ cup fat-free, reduced-sodium honey-mustard salad dressing and 1 cup diced avocado and ½ cup shredded Monterey Jack cheese

COMPLETE MEAL SERVING
506 calories / 14 g total fat / 128 calories from fat / 25% calories from fat
23 mg cholesterol / 651 mg sodium / 71 g carbohydrate / 22 g fiber / 20 g sugars / 26 g protein

moving forward
Write your weight goal and post it where you'll see it every day.

White Bean and Escarole Ragout

Prep Time: 5 minutes ■ Cook Time: 15 minutes

When cooking dark green leafy vegetables such as escarole, kale, collard greens, or chard, use a pair of tongs. They allow you to grab the greens to easily move them around the pan.

8   ounces dried whole grain spaghetti
2   cloves garlic, thinly sliced
1   teaspoon olive oil
1   large head escarole (about 1½ pounds), washed and chopped
½   cup reduced-sodium vegetable broth
1   19-ounce can cannellini beans, rinsed and drained
¼   teaspoon crushed red pepper flakes
¼   teaspoon salt
½   cup grated Parmesan cheese
½   cup pine nuts, toasted

1 Prepare pasta according to package directions. Drain and divide among 4 plates. Meanwhile, in large saucepan cook and stir garlic in hot oil over medium-high heat for 1 minute. Add half the escarole and cook until slightly wilted; add remaining escarole and broth. Cook and stir for 10 minutes or until escarole is wilted and tender. Add beans, red pepper flakes, and salt; cook for 2 minutes, stirring, or until heated through.

2 Divide escarole mixture over the spaghetti; top each plate with 2 tablespoons of the cheese and one-fourth of the pine nuts.

Makes 4 servings

COMPLETE MEAL SERVING
474 calories / 15 g total fat / 133 calories from fat / 27% calories from fat
8 mg cholesterol / 814 mg sodium / 67 g carbohydrate / 17 g fiber / 6 g sugars / 23 g protein

Black Bean and Arugula Burritos

Prep Time: 15 minutes ■ Cook Time: 15 minutes

Arugula, also known as rocket, is an aromatic salad green with a peppery flavor that's common in Italian cooking. Look for it with the bags of salads or loose with the lettuces. Baby arugula is most often packed in bags.

1   cup uncooked quick-cooking brown rice
2   large cloves garlic, minced
1   teaspoon olive oil
2   cups packed baby arugula
1   15-ounce can sodium-free black beans, rinsed and drained
½   cup frozen corn kernels, thawed
4   8-inch whole wheat tortillas
½   cup shredded reduced-fat, reduced-sodium four-cheese Mexican blend
½   cup salsa
½   cup sour cream

1 Prepare rice according to package directions.

2 Meanwhile, in large nonstick skillet cook garlic in hot oil over medium heat for 1 minute. Add arugula and cook for 2 minutes or until wilted. Stir in beans, corn, and rice; heat through.

3 Warm tortillas according to package directions. Divide bean mixture down center of each tortilla. Sprinkle each with 2 tablespoons cheese, 2 tablespoons salsa, and 2 tablespoons sour cream. Fold top and bottom of each tortilla over. Fold one side up and over the filling, rolling until the filling is enclosed.

Makes 4 servings

to complete the meal   For 4 servings: 6 cups lettuce with 1 cup chopped cucumber and 1 cup shredded carrot tossed with ⅓ cup fat-free oil-and-vinegar salad dressing and ½ cup sliced black olives

COMPLETE MEAL SERVING
485 calories / 15 g total fat / 138 calories from fat / 27% calories from fat
23 mg cholesterol / 740 mg sodium / 76 g carbohydrate / 12 g fiber / 9 g sugars / 18 g protein

Florentine Frittata

Prep Time: 10 minutes ■ Cook Time: 18 minutes

Frittatas, Italian-style omelets, have all the ingredients stirred into the eggs rather than on top of the egg mixture as in French omelets. Cooked in the skillet until the eggs are almost set, frittatas finish cooking in the oven.

2	cups egg substitute
½	cup grated Parmesan cheese
½	teaspoon garlic powder
¼	teaspoon ground black pepper
1	cup chopped onion (1 large)
1	teaspoon olive oil
1	16-ounce bag frozen country-style (shredded) hash brown potatoes
1	10-ounce box frozen chopped spinach, thawed and squeezed dry
¼	cup dried tomato halves (not packed in oil), chopped

1 Preheat oven to 400°F.

2 In medium bowl whisk together egg substitute, cheese, garlic powder, and pepper.

3 In large ovenproof nonstick skillet cook and stir onion in hot oil over medium-high heat for 4 minutes or until just tender. Stir in potatoes, spinach, and tomato; cook for 1 minute. Pour in the egg mixture and cook for 3 minutes or until the bottom of the frittata is set.

4 Bake for 10 minutes or until set.

Makes 4 servings

to complete the meal   Per serving: 1 wedge iceberg lettuce (one-sixth of head) and 1 tablespoon sliced black olives with 2 tablespoons fat-free Thousand Island salad dressing and 1 tablespoon flaxseed ■ 1 whole wheat roll with ½ teaspoon trans-fat-free canola margarine

COMPLETE MEAL SERVING
449 calories / 12 g total fat / 112 calories from fat / 25% calories from fat
8 mg cholesterol / 1,063 mg sodium / 58 g carbohydrate / 9 g fiber / 15 g sugars / 27 g protein

Summer Vegetable Quesadillas

Prep Time: 5 minutes ■ Cook Time: 25 minutes

Quesadillas are often appetizers, but here they make a lovely, quick, light meal that's perfect for summer nights. Any prepared hummus will work; use plain or try red pepper, garlic, or scallion flavor.

Nonstick cooking spray
2 zucchini and/or yellow squash (1 pound), cut into ½-inch pieces
1 small eggplant (8 ounces), cut into ½-inch pieces
1 large red onion, cut into ½-inch pieces
¼ cup lemon juice
1 teaspoon olive oil
2 tablespoons snipped fresh oregano
2 tablespoons snipped fresh rosemary
½ teaspoon ground black pepper
12 9-inch whole wheat tortillas
1½ cups prepared hummus

1 Preheat oven to 425°F. Lightly spray jelly-roll pan with nonstick cooking spray.

2 In large bowl combine squash, eggplant, onion, lemon juice, oil, oregano, rosemary, and pepper. Place on prepared pan and roast for 20 minutes or until tender.

3 Lightly spray 3 baking sheets with nonstick cooking spray. Place 2 tortillas on each sheet.

4 Spread ¼ cup of the hummus over each tortilla on baking sheets. Evenly divide vegetables over hummus and top with remaining tortillas. Lightly spray tops with nonstick cooking spray. Bake for 5 minutes or until heated through, turning once.

Makes 6 servings

to complete the meal For 6 servings: 6 cups chopped romaine lettuce tossed with ⅓ cup fat-free ranch dressing and ¼ cup chopped walnuts

COMPLETE MEAL SERVING
406 calories / 14 g total fat / 129 calories from fat / 29% calories from fat
0 mg cholesterol / 659 mg sodium / 64 g carbohydrate / 11 g fiber / 6 g sugars / 14 g protein

Southern Vegetarian Platter

Prep Time: 5 minutes ■ Cook Time: 25 minutes

When cooking hearty greens, washing them well removes any sand or grit. Don't dry the greens after washing because the water that remains on the greens adds moisture during cooking, preventing the greens from sticking and allowing them to steam slightly.

2 pounds sweet potatoes, peeled and cut into 2-inch pieces
1 pound collard greens
1 clove garlic, minced
1 teaspoon olive oil
½ pound asparagus, trimmed and cut into 2-inch pieces
½ pound green beans, trimmed and cut into 2-inch pieces
2 tablespoons maple syrup
½ teaspoon vanilla
¼ teaspoon orange extract
½ cup shredded Monterey Jack cheese
¼ cup chopped pecans

1 In large saucepan bring potato covered with water to boiling over high heat. Reduce heat to medium, cover, and simmer for 15 minutes or until tender. Drain well.

2 Meanwhile, remove and discard collard stems. Coarsely chop leaves.

3 In large skillet cook garlic in hot oil over medium heat for 1 minute. Add collard greens and cook, turning with tongs, for 3 minutes. Add asparagus and green beans; cook and stir for 5 minutes or until vegetables are crisp-tender.

4 In food processor combine potato, maple syrup, vanilla, and orange extract. Process until smooth. Divide among 4 plates. Divide vegetable mixture among plates. Sprinkle vegetables with cheese and pecans.

Makes 4 servings

COMPLETE MEAL SERVING
374 calories / 12 g total fat / 106 calories from fat / 27% calories from fat
13 mg cholesterol / 117 mg sodium / 60 g carbohydrate / 9 g fiber / 29 g sugars / 11 g protein

moving forward
Cook with fresh fruits and vegetables whenever possible. They are full of nutrients and don't come packed in high-calorie sauces.

Millet with a Southern Twist

Prep Time: 10 minutes ■ Cook Time: 20 minutes

Millet, a tiny seed often used in bird seed, is a versatile gluten-free grain. When prepared as described below, it's fluffy like rice. When cooked in four times the amount of water for about 35 minutes, it becomes creamy like mashed potatoes.

3	cups water
1	cup millet
½	cup chopped onion
½	cup chopped carrot (1)
1	teaspoon olive oil
2	cloves garlic, minced
½	teaspoon minced chile pepper (see tip, page 34)
1	large bunch mustard greens
1	19-ounce can white beans, rinsed and drained
½	cup shredded Monterey Jack cheese
½	cup chopped pecans

1 In medium saucepan bring the water to boiling. Add millet and bring to simmer. Cover and simmer for 20 minutes or until tender. Remove from heat and set aside, covered, for 5 minutes or until all the water is absorbed.

2 Meanwhile, in large skillet cook onion and carrot in hot oil over medium heat for 5 minutes or until lightly brown. Add garlic and cook for 1 minute. Place onion mixture in bowl.

3 Add chile pepper and mustard greens to skillet; cook and stir for 5 minutes or until tender. Add beans and cook for 2 minutes to heat through. Divide mustard green mixture among 6 plates.

4 Stir millet and cheese into bowl with onion mixture; toss to blend. Divide among plates with greens. Garnish with pecans.

Makes 6 servings

COMPLETE MEAL SERVING
472 calories / 13 g total fat / 117 calories from fat / 25% calories from fat
8 mg cholesterol / 198 mg sodium / 74 g carbohydrate / 8 g fiber / 3 g sugars / 16 g protein

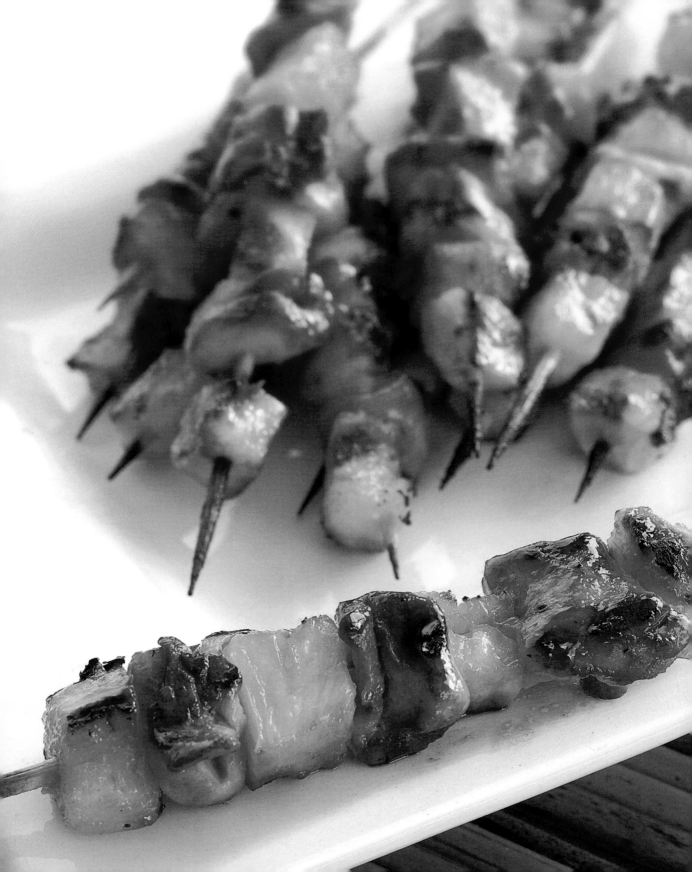

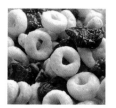

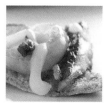

little bites

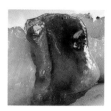

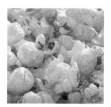

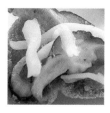

◀ *Pineapple-Chicken Brochettes, page 196*

SNACKS

Nutty Fruit Crisps	187
Chocolate Pecan Roll	187
Maple-Glazed Popcorn	188
Garbanzo Nuts	188
Trail Mix	190
Buffalo-Style Crackers	190
Spicy Tuna Dip	192
Edamame Spread with Sesame Crisps	193
Watermelon-Feta Crostini	194
Crab Bites	194
Creamy Fruit Cup	195
Hot Apple Crunch	195

APPETIZERS

Pineapple-Chicken Brochettes	196
Thai Shrimp Skewers	198
Artichoke Bruschetta	199
Stuffed Mushrooms	200
Black Bean Quesadillas	201
Shiitake-Caramelized Onion Pizzas	202
Garden Vegetable Bruschetta Salad	204
Mini Vegetable Croquettes	205

Nutty Fruit Crisps

Prep Time: 5 minutes

Opting for crispbread with fruits, oats, and honey starts you out with a mouthful of flavor. Spreading the crispbread with nut butter and banana makes this snack a sure winner.

   1   teaspoon soynut butter
   1   whole grain crispbread with fruits, oats, and honey
   ⅓   banana, sliced

Spread thin layer of the soynut butter over the crispbread. Top with banana.

Makes 1 serving

PER SERVING
100 calories / 3 g total fat / 30 calories from fat / 30% calories from fat
0 mg cholesterol / 51 mg sodium / 16 g carbohydrate / 2 g fiber / 7 g sugars / 2 g protein

Chocolate Pecan Roll

Prep Time: 5 minutes ■ Freeze Time: 2 hours

These chocolaty treats keep overindulgence at bay. To save time, make up a batch to keep in the freezer. Store them for up to 2 months. They're great to have on hand for a late-night or last-minute snack.

   1   package 70-calorie chocolate shake mix
   2   tablespoons water
   1½ teaspoons chopped pecans

Mix all ingredients in small bowl. Place on waxed paper or plastic wrap; roll into log. Freeze for 2 hours or until firm.

Makes 1 serving

PER SERVING
95 calories / 3 g total fat / 27 calories from fat / 28% calories from fat
0 mg cholesterol / 32 mg sodium / 10 g carbohydrate / 3 g fiber / 0 g sugars / 7 g protein

Maple-Glazed Popcorn

Prep Time: 4 minutes ■ Cook Time: 5 minutes

Similar to caramel corn, this sweet-and-salty treat makes a delicious snack in midafternoon.

8	cups air-popped popcorn
¼	cup maple syrup
2	tablespoons packed light brown sugar
⅛	teaspoon cinnamon
1½	tablespoons butter

1 Place popcorn in large bowl.

2 In small saucepan stir together syrup, sugar, and cinnamon. Bring to boiling over medium heat. Stir in butter and remove from heat. Pour over popcorn, tossing to coat. Store popcorn in airtight container for up to 4 days.

Makes 6 servings

PER SERVING
103 calories / 3 g total fat / 30 calories from fat / 29% calories from fat
8 mg cholesterol / 25 mg sodium / 18 g carbohydrate / 2 g fiber / 8 g sugars / 1 g protein

Garbanzo Nuts

Prep Time: 5 minutes ■ Bake Time: 20 minutes

To vary the flavor in this snack, use cinnamon instead of the chili powder for a sweeter treat.

	Nonstick cooking spray
2	15-ounce cans garbanzo beans, drained
1	teaspoon olive oil
1	teaspoon chili powder
¼	teaspoon sea salt

1 Preheat oven to 425°F. Lightly spray 15×10×1-inch baking pan with nonstick cooking spray.

2 Pour beans onto paper towel to absorb any extra moisture. Place beans in prepared pan; bake for 10 minutes. Drizzle with oil and chili powder, toss to coat, and spread out on pan. Bake for 10 minutes more or until lightly brown. Sprinkle with sea salt. Cool on rack. Store nuts in airtight container for up to 7 days.

Makes 8 servings

PER SERVING
68 calories / 2 g total fat / 13 calories from fat / 20% calories from fat
0 mg cholesterol / 289 mg sodium / 10 g carbohydrate / 3 g fiber / 1 g sugars / 3 g protein

Maple-Glazed Popcorn ▶

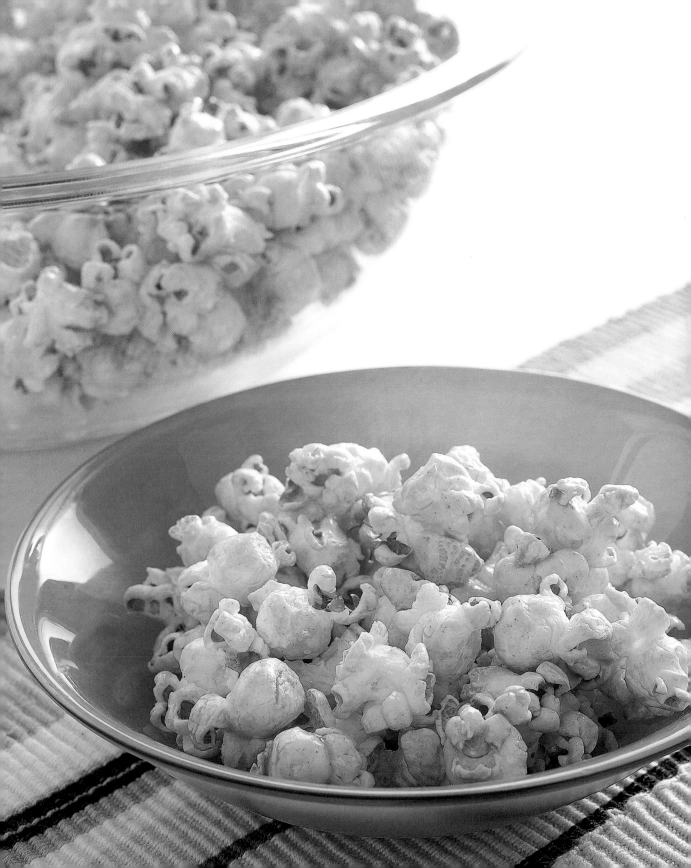

Trail Mix

Prep Time: 5 minutes

Have these bags of sweet tasty treats on hand for a snack to grab and go. To increase the antioxidants in this recipe, opt for chocolate pieces with 50 percent or more cocoa.

- 1 cup toasted honey oat cereal
- ¼ cup dried cherries
- ¼ cup semisweet mini chocolate pieces

1 In medium bowl combine cereal, cherries, and chocolate pieces. Divide mixture among 5 plastic snack bags.

2 Store trail mix in resealable plastic bags for up to 2 weeks.

Makes 5 servings

PER SERVING
100 calories / 3 g total fat / 31 calories from fat / 31% calories from fat
0 mg cholesterol / 50 mg sodium / 17 g carbohydrate / 1 g fiber / 13 g sugars / 2 g protein

Buffalo-Style Crackers

Prep Time: 10 minutes

Creamy, crunchy, and with a spark of fire—these are no ordinary crackers. The combination of flavors and textures comes together in an amazingly simple-but-satisfying snack.

- 6 ounces fat-free cream cheese
- 2 ounces crumbled blue cheese
- 1 dash hot red pepper sauce
- 12 3¾×1¾-inch melba toasts

1 In small bowl using a fork mash cream cheese, blue cheese, and red pepper sauce until smooth.

2 Spoon 2 tablespoons of the cream cheese mixture onto each toast.

3 Store crackers in airtight container in refrigerator for up to 3 days.

Makes 6 servings

PER SERVING
100 calories / 3 g total fat / 31 calories from fat / 31% calories from fat
9 mg cholesterol / 380 mg sodium / 10 g carbohydrate / 1 g fiber / 0 g sugars / 7 g protein

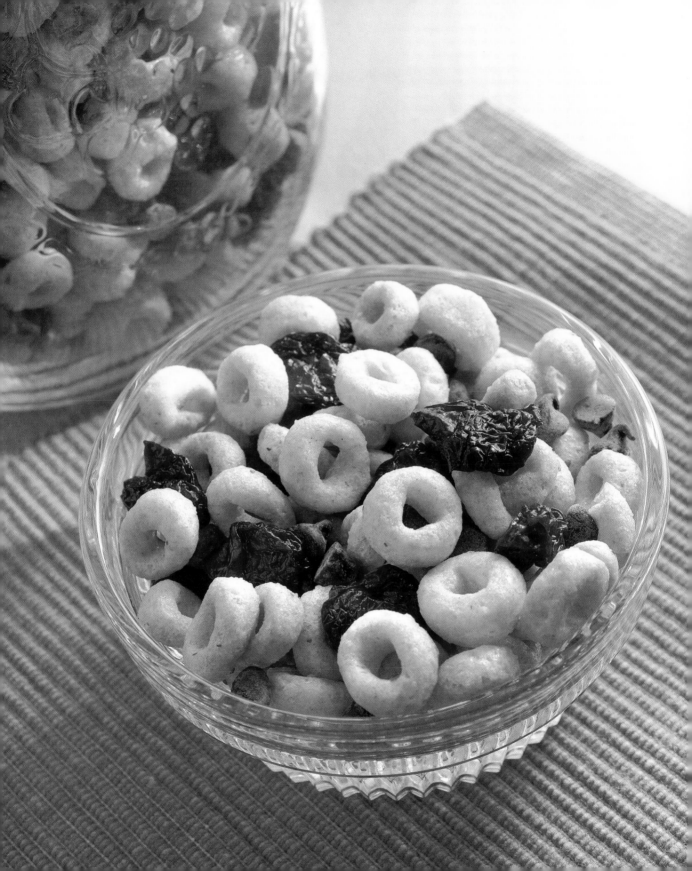

Spicy Tuna Dip

Prep Time: 10 minutes

Paired with an array of colorful veggies, this spicy tuna salad offers enjoyment without a shred of guilt. Packed with protein and omega-3 fatty acids, it's as healthy as it is satisfying.

2	3½-ounce cans tuna fish packed in water, drained
⅔	cup reduced-fat mayonnaise
½	cup snipped fresh cilantro
¼	cup chopped pickled jalapeño pepper
½	cup chopped onion
1	8-ounce can mixed vegetables, drained
1	teaspoon ground white pepper
1	red sweet pepper, cut into 16 strips
2	carrots, cut into 16 strips

1 In medium bowl combine tuna, mayonnaise, cilantro, jalapeño, onion, mixed vegetables, and white pepper.

2 Serve with sweet pepper and carrot strips.

3 Store dip in airtight container and vegetables in resealable plastic bag in refrigerator for up to 4 days.

Makes 8 servings

PER SERVING
99 calories / 3 g total fat / 31 calories from fat / 31% calories from fat
10 mg cholesterol / 378 mg sodium / 10 g carbohydrate / 2 g fiber / 5 g sugars / 7 g protein

moving forward
Sometimes when you think that you are hungry, you may be thirsty. Start with a glass of water.

Edamame Spread with Sesame Crisps

Prep Time: 20 minutes

Edamame (pronounced ed-dah-MAH-meh) is the Japanese name for fresh soybeans. Just ½ cup of this luscious, citrus-flavored legume spread punches up the fiber, protein, and vitamin/mineral content of your daily diet. In fact, 1 serving contains as much fiber as 4 slices of whole wheat bread. When choosing a meal to pair with this recipe, choose one that is not prepared with oil.

2	cups frozen shelled edamame
2	large cloves garlic
1	teaspoon grated lime zest
1	to 2 tablespoons lime juice
1	teaspoon olive oil
½	teaspoon salt
¼	teaspoon ground black pepper
¼	cup water
18	sesame rice crackers

1 In medium saucepan of boiling water cook edamame and garlic for 5 minutes or until tender. Drain, reserving ¼ cup water.

2 In food processor or blender puree edamame, garlic, zest, lime juice, oil, salt, pepper, and the water for 2 minutes or until very smooth, scraping sides of bowl.

3 Serve with crackers.

4 Store spread in airtight container in refrigerator for up to 4 days.

Makes 6 servings

PER SERVING
97 calories / 3 g total fat / 25 calories from fat / 26% calories from fat
0 mg cholesterol / 244 mg sodium / 11 g carbohydrate / 3 g fiber / 1 g sugars / 6 g protein

Watermelon-Feta Crostini

Prep Time: 10 minutes ■ Cook Time: 3 minutes

If you can't get to the grill for this summer treat, you can broil the bread for 4 minutes or until toasted, turning once.

3½	ounces feta cheese
½	cup loosely packed snipped fresh mint
	Nonstick grilling spray
8	1-inch-thick slices whole wheat Italian bread
8	ounces watermelon, cut into 8 thin slices

1 In small bowl using a fork whip cheese until fluffy. Stir in mint.

2 Lightly spray grill grate with nonstick grilling spray. Preheat grill to medium heat. Grill bread for 3 minutes or until brown, turning once.

3 Spread cheese mixture over bread slices. Top with watermelon. To store, wrap separately in foil and refrigerate for up to 2 days.

Makes 8 servings

PER SERVING
99 calories / 3 g total fat / 30 calories from fat / 30% calories from fat
11 mg cholesterol / 257 mg sodium / 14 g carbohydrate / 1 g fiber / 3 g sugars / 4 g protein

Crab Bites

Prep Time: 10 minutes

There's no need to throw a party to treat yourself to this easy and elegant snack.

1	6½-ounce can crabmeat, drained and flaked
½	cup fat-free cream cheese, room temperature
¼	cup finely snipped fresh chives
4	3¾×1¾ ×⅛-inch slices whole wheat melba toasts

In small bowl using a fork blend crabmeat, cheese, and chives. Divide mixture among melba toasts. Store dip in airtight container in refrigerator and melba toasts in resealable plastic bag for up to 3 days.

Makes 4 servings

PER SERVING
91 calories / 1 g total fat / 10 calories from fat / 11% calories from fat
35 mg cholesterol / 368 mg sodium / 6 g carbohydrate / 0 g fiber / 0 g sugars / 15 g protein

Creamy Fruit Cup

Prep Time: 5 minutes

Ricotta cheese is a natural for sweet dishes—think cannoli. Here it's studded with the tropical flavors of pineapple and banana. For pizzazz sprinkle with a pinch of ground ginger, nutmeg, or cinnamon.

¼ cup crushed pineapple packed in juice, undrained
1½ tablespoons part-skim ricotta cheese
¼ small banana, chopped

In small bowl stir together pineapple and ricotta cheese. Fold in banana.

Makes 1 serving

PER SERVING
98 calories / 3 g total fat / 28 calories from fat / 29% calories from fat
12 mg cholesterol / 25 mg sodium / 15 g carbohydrate / 1 g fiber / 11 g sugars / 3 g protein

Hot Apple Crunch

Prep Time: 5 minutes ■ Cook Time: 3 minutes

Tender apple pieces come to life when tossed with cinnamon sugar and drizzled with vanilla yogurt. For crunch chopped pecans finish off the treat.

1 small apple, cut into ½-inch pieces
2 tablespoons water
½ teaspoon cinnamon sugar
1 tablespoon vanilla yogurt
1½ teaspoons chopped pecans

1 Place apple, the water, and cinnamon sugar in small microwave-safe bowl. Cover with microwave-safe plastic wrap, vented on one side. Microwave on 100% power (high) for 3 minutes. Let cool 1 minute.

2 Spoon apple mixture into dessert dish and drizzle with yogurt. Sprinkle with pecans.

Makes 1 serving

PER SERVING
104 calories / 3 g total fat / 30 calories from fat / 29% calories from fat
2 mg cholesterol / 11 mg sodium / 19 g carbohydrate / 3 g fiber / 15 g sugars / 1 g protein

Pineapple-Chicken Brochettes

Prep Time: 25 minutes ■ Cook Time: 5 minutes

Slightly frozen chicken cuts quickly and easily: Place raw chicken in the freezer for 20 minutes before cutting it into bite-size pieces. Tip: A ¾-inch cube is roughly the size of a grape. To keep your daily oil consumption down, have this appetizer with a meal that contains no oil.

12	6-inch bamboo skewers
3	tablespoons reduced-sodium soy sauce
2	tablespoons plum preserves
1	teaspoon toasted sesame oil
¼	cup fat-free, reduced-sodium chicken broth
1	teaspoon grated fresh ginger
2	cloves garlic, minced
1	pound skinless, boneless chicken breast, cut into 36 ¾-inch cubes
1	20-ounce can pineapple chunks in juice, drained

1 Soak bamboo skewers in water for 30 minutes.

2 In medium bowl combine soy sauce, preserves, oil, broth, ginger, and garlic. Add chicken; toss to coat. Let stand at room temperature for 20 minutes.

3 Preheat broiler.

4 Alternately thread 3 chicken pieces and 4 pineapple chunks onto each bamboo skewer. Brush with remaining marinade. Place skewers on rack in broiler pan. Cover exposed parts of bamboo with foil.

5 Broil 5 inches from heat for 5 minutes or until chicken is brown and no longer pink, turning once.

6 Store in airtight container in refrigerator for up to 4 days.

Makes 12 servings

PER SERVING
74 calories / 1 g total fat / 12 calories from fat / 16% calories from fat
21 mg cholesterol / 183 mg sodium / 7 g carbohydrate / 0 g fiber / 6 g sugars / 8 g protein

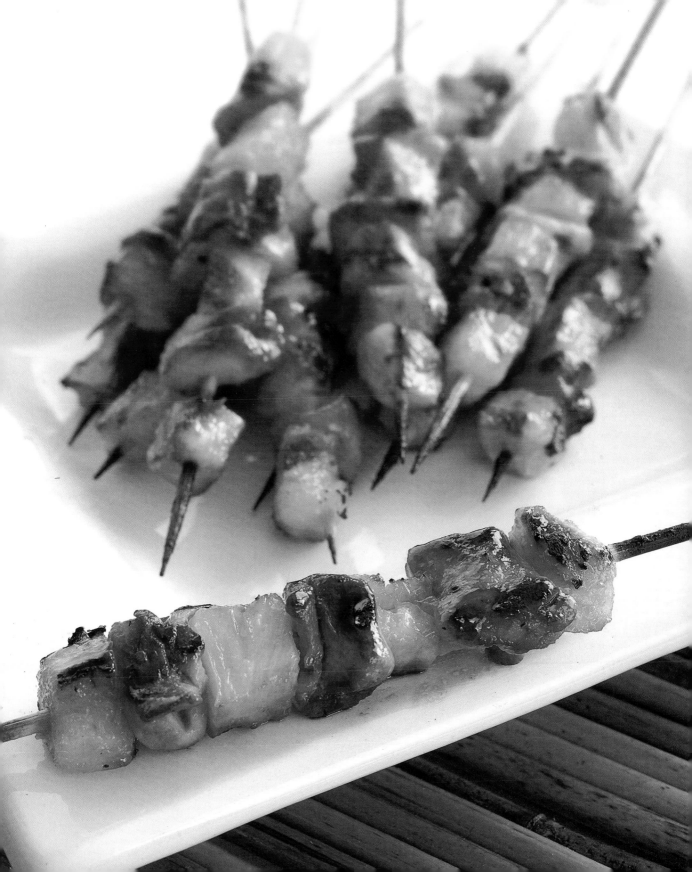

Thai Shrimp Skewers

Prep Time: 10 minutes ■ Cook Time: 5 minutes

Although the presentation is lovely with the shrimp threaded onto skewers, you can serve this zesty appetizer on plates instead. These protein-rich bites are a great way to start a meal because they'll keep you from getting too hungry and overeating at the meal. Pair this with a meal that does not contain any oil.

- 1 clove garlic, minced
- 1 teaspoon toasted sesame oil
- 2 teaspoons water
- ½ cup lime juice
- 2 tablespoons sugar
- 2 tablespoons fish sauce
- ½ teaspoon Vietnamese chili paste
- 1 pound peeled and deveined medium shrimp
- 8 6-inch bamboo skewers
- 4 teaspoons sesame seeds
- ½ cup loosely packed coarsely snipped fresh cilantro

1 In large nonstick skillet cook garlic in hot oil for 1 minute over medium heat. Add the water, lime juice, sugar, fish sauce, and chili paste. Bring to boiling. Add shrimp and cook for 4 minutes or until shrimp are opaque. With slotted spoon remove shrimp to plate. Thread shrimp onto eight 6-inch bamboo skewers. Place 1 skewer on each of 8 plates. Sprinkle with the sesame seeds.

2 Stir cilantro into sauce. Divide sauce into 8 ramekins or small bowls; place 1 ramekin on each plate.

3 Store shrimp and sauce in airtight container in refrigerator for up to 4 days.

Makes 8 servings

PER SERVING
61 calories / 2 g total fat / 15 calories from fat / 25% calories from fat
84 mg cholesterol / 129 mg sodium / 2 g carbohydrate / 0 g fiber / 1 g sugars / 9 g protein

Artichoke Bruschetta

Prep Time: 15 minutes ■ Cook Time: 11 minutes

In Italy polenta was once a symbol of poverty, a simple food that sustained and soothed. Despite its humble beginnings, polenta is now as mainstream as pizza and pasta. Look for convenient ready-to-slice tubes in the refrigerated section of the supermarket. This dish works with almost any main dish; just choose one that does not contain oil in the recipe.

1	clove garlic, minced
1	teaspoon olive oil
1	9-ounce box frozen artichoke hearts, thawed
2	tomatoes, seeded and chopped
1	tablespoon prepared pesto
¼	cup white wine
1	tablespoon lemon juice
1	1-pound tube polenta, cut into 8 slices
2	tablespoons grated Parmesan cheese

1 Preheat broiler.

2 In medium nonstick skillet cook garlic in hot oil for 1 minute over medium heat. Add artichoke hearts and their liquid, tomato, pesto, and wine. Cook, stirring constantly, for 4 minutes or until wine evaporates and tomato breaks down. Stir in lemon juice; remove from heat.

3 Place polenta on broiler pan and broil 4 inches from heat for 5 minutes or until brown, turning once. Top with artichoke mixture. Broil for 1 minute or until lightly brown. Remove from oven; sprinkle with cheese.

4 Store bruschetta in airtight container in refrigerator for up to 4 days.

Makes 8 servings

PER SERVING
81 calories / 2 g total fat / 20 calories from fat / 23% calories from fat
2 mg cholesterol / 233 mg sodium / 13 g carbohydrate / 3 g fiber / 2 g sugars / 3 g protein

Stuffed Mushrooms

Prep Time: 10 minutes ■ Cook Time: 10 minutes

The mild, earthy flavor of the mushrooms provides a perfect foundation for the lightly seasoned chicken filling. Before use, mushrooms should be wiped with a damp paper towel or, if necessary, rinsed with cold water and dried thoroughly.

　　　Nonstick cooking spray
6　ounces ground, skinless, boneless chicken breast
¼　cup chopped onion
2　tablespoons panko (Japanese bread crumbs)
1　clove garlic, minced
2　tablespoons snipped fresh flat-leaf parsley
1　egg white
1　tablespoon Dijon mustard
4　teaspoons reduced-fat mayonnaise
2　teaspoons Worcestershire sauce
12　large white mushrooms, stems removed

1 Preheat oven to 450°F. Lightly spray 15×10×1-inch baking pan with nonstick cooking spray.

2 In small bowl combine chicken, onion, panko, garlic, parsley, egg white, mustard, mayonnaise, and Worcestershire sauce. Divide chicken mixture among mushrooms. Place mushrooms, filled sides up, on prepared pan.

3 Bake for 10 minutes or until tops are light brown and chicken is no longer pink.

4 Store mushrooms in airtight container in refrigerator for up to 4 days.

Makes 4 servings

PER SERVING
98 calories / 3 g total fat / 30 calories from fat / 31% calories from fat
24 mg cholesterol / 166 mg sodium / 8 g carbohydrate / 0 g fiber / 2 g sugars / 10 g protein

Black Bean Quesadillas

Prep Time: 10 minutes ■ Cook Time: 15 minutes

Mashed beans studded with salsa and avocado make a delicious filling for whole wheat tortillas. Turning the tortillas allows for both sides to brown. For easy turning use two spatulas, one on either side.

Nonstick cooking spray
4   6-inch whole wheat flour tortillas
1   cup canned black beans, rinsed and drained
1   cup salsa
2   tablespoons reduced-fat sour cream
½   avocado, halved, pitted, peeled, and very thinly sliced

1 Preheat oven to 375°F. Lightly spray baking sheet with nonstick cooking spray. Place 2 tortillas on sheet.

2 In medium bowl using potato masher coarsely mash beans. Stir in salsa and sour cream. Spread bean mixture evenly on tortillas on baking sheet. Top evenly with avocado. Place remaining 2 tortillas over avocado. Spray tops with nonstick cooking spray. Bake for 15 minutes or until heated through, turning once.

3 Store quesadillas in airtight container in refrigerator for up to 4 days.

Makes 8 servings

PER SERVING
101 calories / 3 g total fat / 30 calories from fat / 30% calories from fat
1 mg cholesterol / 294 mg sodium / 16 g carbohydrate / 3 g fiber / 2 g sugars / 3 g protein

moving forward

Join a class that interests you at your gym. You'll burn calories, build muscle, and be motivated by working out with other people.

Shiitake-Caramelized Onion Pizzas

Prep Time: 5 minutes ■ Cook Time: 15 minutes

With a bit of time and patience but very little work, caramelizing turns a tearjerker onion into a sweet delicacy. Breaking down and browning the natural sugars in the onion gives it a melt-in-your-mouth texture and rich, savory flavor. Shopping tip: The flatter the onion, the sweeter it will be. When serving these with lunch or dinner, choose a main dish that does not contain any oil.

1	medium sweet onion, sliced and separated into rings
1	teaspoon olive oil
1	teaspoon water
6	ounces shiitake mushrooms, stemmed and sliced
⅛	teaspoon salt
2	6-inch whole wheat pita breads
½	cup shredded reduced-fat mozzarella cheese

1 In medium nonstick skillet cook onion in hot oil and the water over medium heat for 10 minutes, stirring occasionally. Add mushrooms and salt; cook for 5 minutes, stirring often.

2 Meanwhile, preheat oven to 425°F. Split each pita bread around edge with knife to make two rounds. Place rounds, cut sides up, on ungreased baking sheet; bake for 5 minutes or just until warm.

3 Divide onion mixture over rounds; sprinkle with cheese. Cut each round into 8 wedges.

4 Store pizzas in airtight container in refrigerator for up to 4 days.

Makes 8 servings

PER SERVING
82 calories / 2 g total fat / 20 calories from fat / 23% calories from fat
3 mg cholesterol / 173 mg sodium / 13 g carbohydrate / 2 g fiber / 1 g sugars / 4 g protein

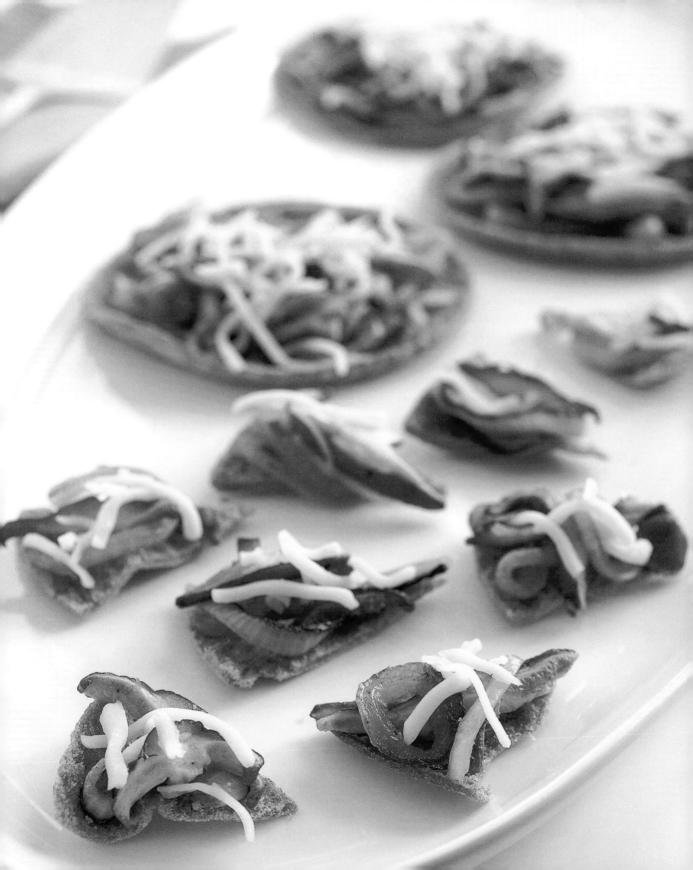

Garden Vegetable Bruschetta Salad

Prep Time: 10 minutes

You can't go wrong with a salad that includes the traditional Italian trio of tomatoes, fresh mozzarella, and fresh basil. To amplify the flavor of a tomato, after slicing it sprinkle slices with salt and allow them to rest for about 5 minutes. Your salad will taste magnifico.

- 3 cups torn lettuce
- 2 medium tomatoes, cut into 3 slices each
- 6 slices fresh mozzarella cheese (3 ounces)
- ½ cup chopped red onion
- 1 large cucumber, seeded and chopped
- ½ cup fat-free Italian vinaigrette
- 6 fresh basil leaves

1 Place ½ cup lettuce on each of 6 small plates; top each with tomato slice. Divide cheese, onion, and cucumber among sliced tomatoes. Drizzle each with 1 tablespoon plus 1 teaspoon dressing; top with basil leaf.

2 Store salad in airtight container in refrigerator for up to 4 days.

Makes 6 servings

PER SERVING
91 calories / 3 g total fat / 26 calories from fat / 29% calories from fat
10 mg cholesterol / 191 mg sodium / 11 g carbohydrate / 2 g fiber / 6 g sugars / 5 g protein

Mini Vegetable Croquettes

Prep Time: 5 minutes ■ Cook Time: 17 minutes

Traditionally croquettes are bound with a rich, high-fat white sauce and then fried. This more healthful version uses lentils to bind and add flavor and texture to the croquettes. Instead of deep-frying, you quickly saute the patties and then bake the croquettes for a crispy finish. For best results, pair this appetizer with a main dish that does not contain any oil.

	Nonstick cooking spray
1	15-ounce can lentils, rinsed and drained
¾	cup fresh bread crumbs
¼	cup finely chopped red sweet pepper
¼	cup finely chopped green sweet pepper
1	clove garlic, minced
½	teaspoon salt
¼	teaspoon ground black pepper
1	teaspoon olive oil
1	teaspoon water

1 Preheat oven to 350°F. Lightly spray baking sheet with nonstick cooking spray.

2 In large bowl with potato masher mash lentils. Stir in bread crumbs, sweet peppers, garlic, salt, and black pepper. Shape into 8 patties.

3 In large nonstick skillet cook patties in hot oil and the water over medium-high heat for 2 minutes or until brown, turning once. Remove to prepared baking sheet.

4 Bake patties for 15 minutes or until heated through.

5 Store croquettes in airtight container in refrigerator for up to 4 days.

Makes 8 servings

PER SERVING
47 calories / 1 g total fat / 7 calories from fat / 14% calories from fat
0 mg cholesterol / 209 mg sodium / 8 g carbohydrate / 3 g fiber / 1 g sugars / 3 g protein

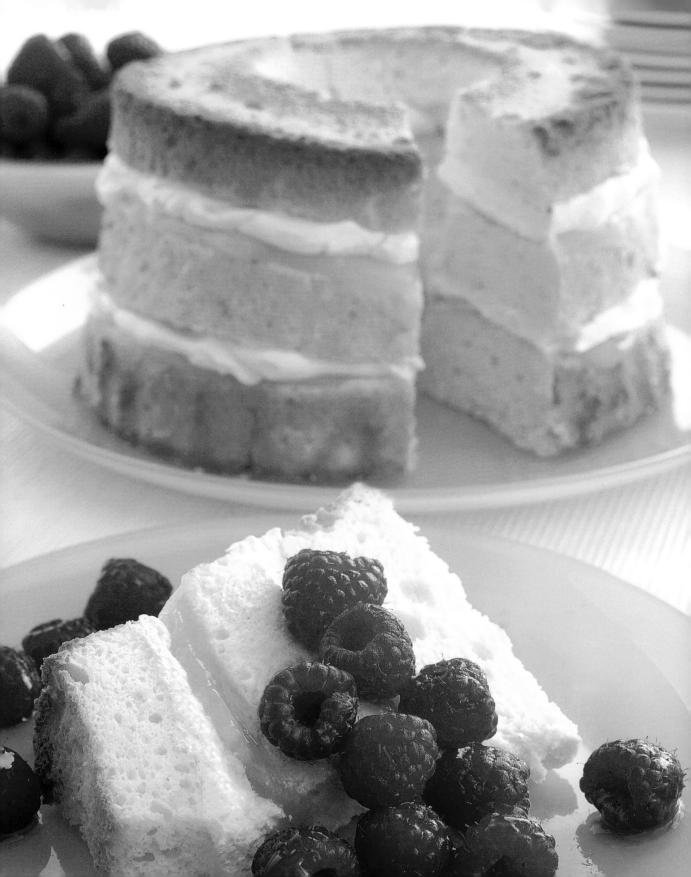

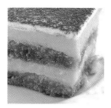

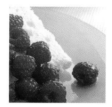

desserts

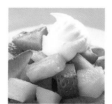

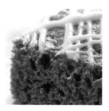

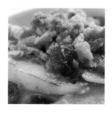

◀ *Lemon Angel Cake with*
Raspberry Syrup, page 228

PUDDINGS, PARFAITS, AND MORE

FROM THE ORCHARD

FROZEN TREATS

BAKED DESSERTS

Chocolate-Banana Trifle

Prep Time: 8 minutes

So rich and sweet, this chocolate-vanilla dessert is sure to please. For a really chocolaty dessert, use the chocolate pudding.

- 1   3.4-ounce box chocolate or vanilla instant pudding mix
- 2   cups cold fat-free (skim) milk
- 6   ounces all-butter pound cake, thawed, if frozen, and cut into bite-size cubes
- 1   small banana, thinly sliced
- 2   tablespoons chocolate syrup

1 Prepare pudding with milk according to package directions.

2 Layer half of the cake cubes in bottom of medium bowl or baking dish. Cover with half of the banana slices, then half of the pudding. Drizzle with half of the syrup.

3 Repeat layers with remaining ingredients. Serve at once or cover and refrigerate for up to 2 days.

Makes twelve ⅓-cup servings

PER SERVING
115 calories / 3 g total fat / 27 calories from fat / 23% calories from fat
32 mg cholesterol / 191 mg sodium / 20 g carbohydrate / 1 g fiber / 14 g sugars / 3 g protein

moving forward
If you're tempted to cheat, think about how many hours of exercise it will take to burn off the extra calories.

Mocha Pudding

Prep Time: 10 minutes ■ Cook Time: 8 minutes

The rich blend of coffee and chocolate is an all-time favorite.

- 1 cup brewed coffee
- ¾ cup fat-free (skim) milk
- 1 3.4-ounce box chocolate pudding mix
- 1 teaspoon vanilla
- ½ cup whipped cream (from pressurized can)
- 4 teaspoons sliced almonds

1 In small saucepan combine coffee and milk. Stir in pudding mix. Cook, stirring often, over medium heat for 5 to 8 minutes or until mixture comes to a boil. Remove from heat and stir in vanilla.

2 Pour pudding into 4 dessert cups. Top each with 2 tablespoons whipped cream and 1 teaspoon almonds.

Makes 4 servings

PER SERVING
141 calories / 3 g total fat / 29 calories from fat / 21% calories from fat
7 mg cholesterol / 375 mg sodium / 25 g carbohydrate / 1 g fiber / 16 g sugars / 3 g protein

Espresso Jelly

Cook Time: 10 minutes ■ Chill Time: 3 hours

This is the perfect way to use leftover coffee or a great excuse to brew a pot of your favorite joe.

- 4 cups very strong coffee
- ¼ cup sugar
- 2 ¼-ounce envelopes gelatin
- ¾ cup nondairy frozen whipped topping, thawed

1 In medium saucepan bring 3¾ cups of the coffee and sugar to boiling. Meanwhile, in small bowl place remaining ¼ cup coffee. Sprinkle gelatin over coffee and let sit for 1 minute or until dissolved. Add gelatin mixture to hot coffee mixture; stir until incorporated. Remove from heat and let cool for 5 minutes.

2 Pour into 4 large bowls or glasses (2 cups each) and refrigerate until firm, about 3 hours. Top each glass with 3 tablespoons of the whipped topping.

Makes 4 servings

PER SERVING
100 calories / 2 g total fat / 21 calories from fat / 21% calories from fat
0 mg cholesterol / 12 mg sodium / 16 g carbohydrate / 0 g fiber / 14 g sugars / 3 g protein

Butterscotch Fondue

Prep Time: 10 minutes ■ Cook Time: 3 minutes

Because this recipe makes eight servings, you may not eat all the fondue in one sitting. To reheat, microwave the fondue on 50% power (medium) for about 30 seconds, stirring once or twice. Or reheat in a small skillet over medium-low heat for 1 to 2 minutes, stirring occasionally.

¾ cup plus 2 tablespoons packed brown sugar
½ cup half-and-half
1 tablespoon butter
1 banana
1 medium apple
2 slices angel food cake ($^1/_{12}$ of 10-inch cake)

1 In small saucepan combine brown sugar, half-and-half, and butter over medium-low heat. Cook, stirring occasionally, for 3 minutes or until sugar dissolves, fondue sauce is slightly thickened, and mixture just barely comes to boiling. Let cool for a few minutes.

2 Meanwhile, cut banana into 16 slices. Halve and core apple; cut into 16 slices. Cut angel food cake into 16 small cubes.

3 Pour warm fondue into small bowl and place bowl on larger plate. Surround bowl with banana slices, apple slices, and cake. Use forks or toothpicks for dipping. (Each serving is scant 2 tablespoons fondue, 2 banana slices, 2 apple slices, and 2 small cubes angel food cake.)

Makes 8 servings

PER SERVING
151 calories / 3 g total fat / 28 calories from fat / 19% calories from fat
9 mg cholesterol / 116 mg sodium / 30 g carbohydrate / 1 g fiber / 27 g sugars / 1 g protein

Tiramisu

Prep Time: 5 minutes ■ Cook Time: 15 minutes

Coffee-soaked ladyfingers topped with a flavorful, rich filling star in this tiramisu that comes together in minutes thanks to pudding mix and prepared ladyfingers. If time permits, prepare it ahead to allow the flavors to mingle. Cover and refrigerate for up to 2 days.

2	3.125-ounce boxes tiramisu or vanilla flavor pudding mix
1	quart reduced-fat (2%) milk
⅔	cup fat-free whipped cream (from pressurized can)
12	ladyfinger cakes (3 ounces), split
½	cup brewed coffee
2	teaspoons unsweetened cocoa powder
1	teaspoon sugar

1 Prepare pudding mix according to package directions using milk. Set aside to cool slightly.

2 In small bowl beat cream with electric mixer on medium speed until soft peaks form.

3 Arrange half of the ladyfingers on bottom of medium baking dish or loaf pan. Sprinkle with half of the coffee. Top with half of the pudding.

4 Place remaining ladyfingers over pudding and sprinkle with remaining coffee. Top with remaining pudding; spread whipped cream over pudding.

5 In small cup combine cocoa powder and sugar. Sprinkle evenly over cream.

6 Refrigerate tiramisu for up to 2 days. Serve cold.

Makes 12 servings

PER SERVING
130 calories / 3 g total fat / 23 calories from fat / 18% calories from fat
33 mg cholesterol / 158 mg sodium / 23 g carbohydrate / 0 g fiber / 16 g sugars / 4 g protein

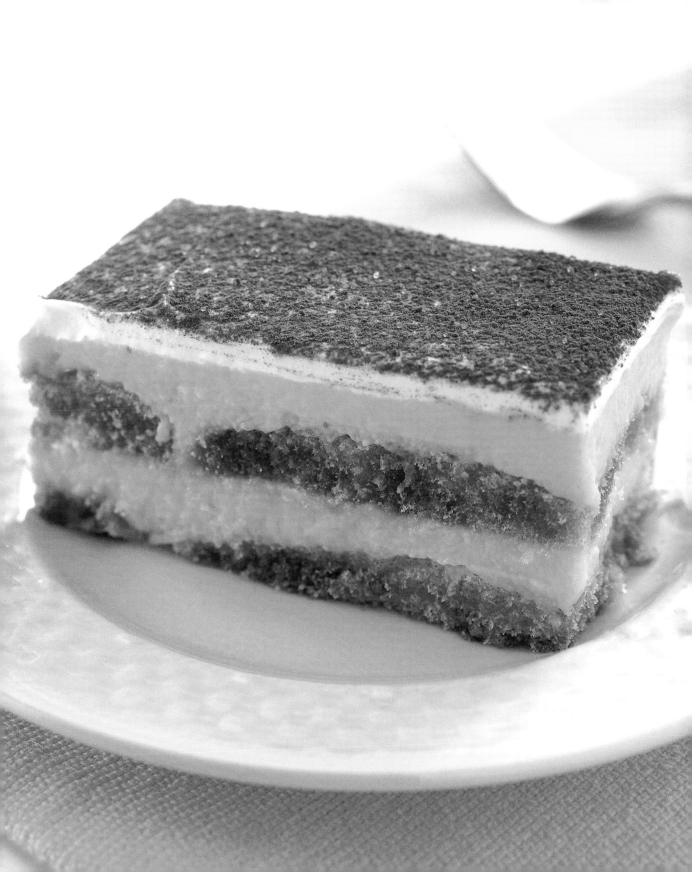

Lemon Cheesecake Parfait

Prep Time: 5 minutes

These light, creamy treats come together in minutes, but if you'd like to prepare them ahead, they can be refrigerated up to 1 hour—any longer and the crumbs will become soft.

4	sheets original-flavor graham crackers (16 crackers)
½	cup part-skim ricotta cheese
2	tablespoons fat-free cream cheese (1 ounce)
2	tablespoons sugar
1	6-ounce container fat-free lemon yogurt

1 Place graham crackers in small resealable plastic bag and seal. With palm of your hand or rolling pin, crush crackers to fine crumbs. Set aside.

2 In blender puree ricotta cheese, cream cheese, and sugar for 1 minute or until very smooth. Add yogurt and gently incorporate with 3 or 4 on-off (pulsing) motions. (Do not overmix or yogurt will liquefy.)

3 In 4 dessert cups or glasses alternate 1 teaspoon of the graham cracker crumbs, scant ¼ cup of the cheese mixture, another 1 teaspoon of the crumbs, and another scant ¼ cup cheese mixture. Top with 1 teaspoon of the crumbs.

Makes 4 servings

PER SERVING
142 calories / 3 g total fat / 30 calories from fat / 21% calories from fat
11 mg cholesterol / 150 mg sodium / 21 g carbohydrate / 0 g fiber / 16 g sugars / 7 g protein

Strawberries with Cannoli Cream

Prep Time: 10 minutes

Rich and sweet, this cream is similar to the kind used to fill cannoli shells. For a more healthful treat, serve it over delicious fresh strawberries. The cream is especially good when very cold; if time permits make it ahead and chill up to 24 hours.

2	tablespoons semisweet chocolate pieces
1	cup reduced-fat ricotta cheese
½	cup powdered sugar
1½	tablespoons fat-free cream cheese
¼	teaspoon vanilla
4	cups sliced strawberries

1 In food processor pulse chocolate chips with on-off motions for 30 seconds or until finely chopped. Place in small bowl.

2 Add ricotta cheese, powdered sugar, cream cheese, and vanilla to food processor. Pulse for 1 minute or until very smooth. Stir into chocolate.

3 Divide strawberries among 6 dessert cups. Spoon about ¼ cup of the cannoli cream over strawberries in each dish.

Makes 6 servings

PER SERVING
141 calories / 3 g total fat / 29 calories from fat / 20% calories from fat
10 mg cholesterol / 58 mg sodium / 25 g carbohydrate / 3 g fiber / 20 g sugars / 5 g protein

moving forward
Low-fat doesn't mean guilt-free. Often fat-free can still be high in calories.

Roasted Summer Fruit Kabobs

Prep Time: 5 minutes ■ Cook Time: 3 minutes

When cooking on wooden skewers, always soak them in water for at least 30 minutes to prevent burning.

2	plums, cut into 6 thick slices
1	peach, cut into 6 thick slices
1	nectarine, cut into 6 thick slices
½	teaspoon ground cinnamon
¼	teaspoon ground nutmeg
1½	cups 2% light vanilla ice cream

1 Lightly spray grill grate or broiler pan with grilling or nonstick cooking spray. Preheat grill or broiler. Alternately thread plum, peach, and nectarine slices onto skewers. Sprinkle with cinnamon and nutmeg.

2 Grill fruit for 3 minutes or until golden, turning once. Divide among 6 dessert dishes. Divide ice cream over fruit.

Makes 6 servings

PER SERVING
97 calories / 2 g total fat / 20 calories from fat / 21% calories from fat
15 mg cholesterol / 33 mg sodium / 18 g carbohydrate / 1 g fiber / 13 g sugars / 2 g protein

Pears with Maple Crème

Prep Time: 10 minutes

On a cold day you can steam the pear halves for 5 minutes, then slice. Serve them warm with the sauce.

½	cup fat-free large-curd cottage cheese
2	tablespoons low-fat maple-flavored yogurt
2	tablespoons maple syrup
3	small ripe Bosc pears
¼	cup walnut halves, finely chopped

1 In blender combine cottage cheese, yogurt, and maple syrup. Process for 1 to 2 minutes or until very smooth.

2 Halve, core, and thinly slice pears. Divide pears among 6 dessert dishes. Divide maple crème over pears. Divide walnuts over the crème.

Makes 6 servings

PER SERVING
105 calories / 3 g total fat / 27 calories from fat / 26% calories from fat
2 mg cholesterol / 7 mg sodium / 17 g carbohydrate / 2 g fiber / 12 g sugars / 4 g protein

Roasted Summer Fruit Kabobs ▶

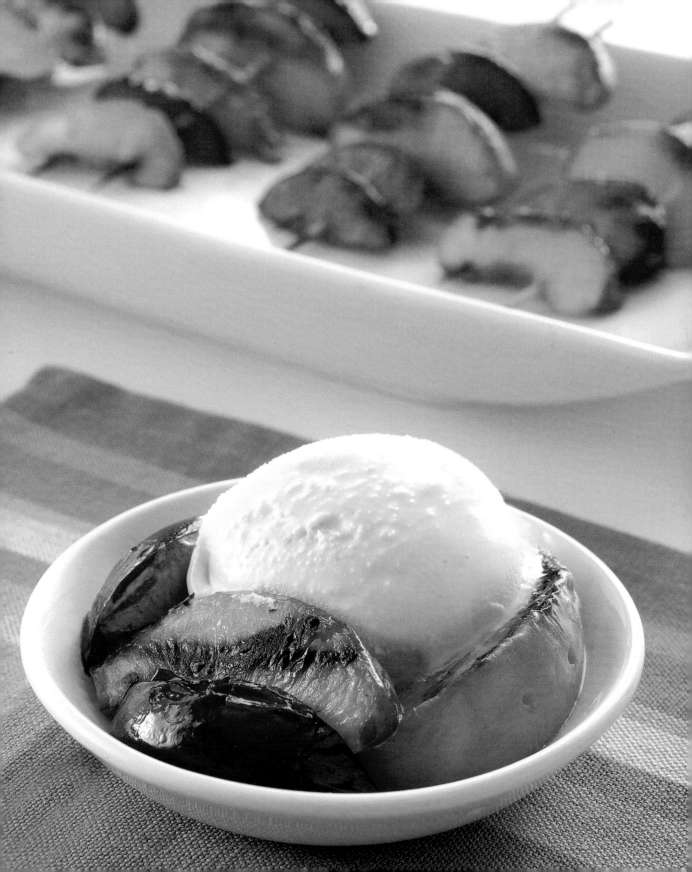

Oranges in Spiced Red Wine

Prep Time: 5 minutes ■ Cook Time: 15 minutes

The oranges and wine are delicious at room temperature, but they can be chilled for use later. Store in an airtight container for up to 2 days.

½	cup dry red wine
⅓	cup sugar
6	whole cloves, slightly crushed
3	navel oranges
1½	cups Greek-style low-fat yogurt
2	tablespoons finely chopped walnuts

1 In small saucepan combine wine, sugar, and cloves over medium-low heat. Bring to boiling. Reduce heat to low; simmer for 15 minutes. Strain through wire-mesh sieve into small bowl. Discard cloves. Set syrup aside to cool slightly.

2 Meanwhile, with paring knife remove peel and bitter white pith from oranges. Over medium bowl section oranges, catching juice and orange sections in bowl. Stir wine syrup into oranges.

3 To serve, divide oranges with syrup among 6 dessert cups. Top each with ¼ cup yogurt and 1 teaspoon walnuts.

Makes 6 servings

PER SERVING
142 calories / 3 g total fat / 25 calories from fat / 18% calories from fat
3 mg cholesterol / 22 mg sodium / 23 g carbohydrate / 2 g fiber / 18 g sugars / 5 g protein

Melon Fans with Strawberry Salsa

Prep Time: 15 minutes

Healthful fruit is a great way to turn frozen yogurt into a guilt-free dessert. Here strawberries, grapes, and banana become a salsa, which is delicious over cantaloupe and frozen yogurt.

- 12 ounces strawberries, hulled
- 1 cup seedless green grapes
- 1 banana, cut into large chunks
- 1 cantaloupe
- 4 cups low-fat vanilla frozen yogurt
- 8 teaspoons slivered almonds, toasted and chopped

1 In food processor combine strawberries, grapes, and banana. With on-off (pulsing) motion process gently to finely chop, scraping down sides of bowl as necessary.

2 Halve cantaloupe. Scoop out seeds. Cut each half into quarters. Thinly slice each quarter and cut off rind. Arrange slices in overlapping, fanlike design on 8 dessert plates. Top each with about ⅓ cup strawberry salsa and ½ cup of the frozen yogurt. Dust with almonds.

Makes 8 servings

PER SERVING
179 calories / 3 g total fat / 25 calories from fat / 14% calories from fat
5 mg cholesterol / 71 mg sodium / 35 g carbohydrate / 31 g fiber / 6 g sugars / 6 g protein

Waffles with Tropical Fruit

Prep Time: 10 minutes

When fruits are tossed with sugar, or macerated, they release their juices, creating a natural syrup. Besides sugar, liqueur or spirits such as brandy may be used to macerate fruits.

2	cups sliced strawberries
1	cup pineapple chunks, chopped
1	cup cubed mango
½	teaspoon sugar
6	whole wheat frozen waffles
6	tablespoons fat-free non-dairy frozen whipped topping, thawed

1 In small bowl combine strawberries, pineapple, mango, and sugar; toss gently. Set aside.

2 Toast waffles.

3 To assemble, place waffles on 6 dessert plates. Spoon about ½ cup of the fruit mixture over each waffle. Top each with 1 tablespoon of the whipped topping.

Makes 6 servings

PER SERVING
147 calories / 3 g total fat / 29 calories from fat / 20% calories from fat
0 mg cholesterol / 214 mg sodium / 28 g carbohydrate / 3 g fiber / 11 g sugars / 3 g protein

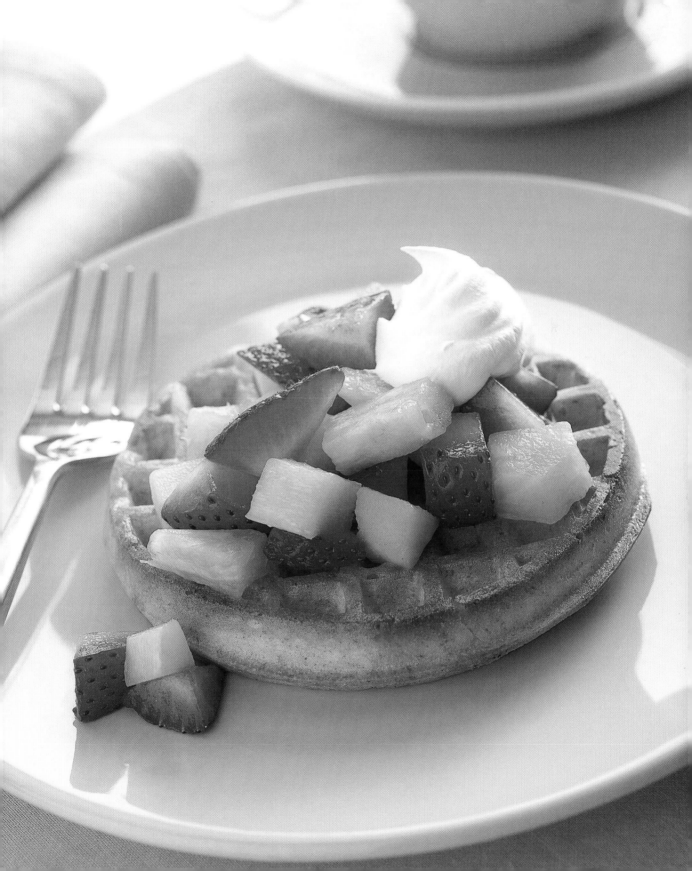

Fruit Salad with Frozen Yogurt

Prep Time: 15 minutes

Not only delicious, this salad is bursting with antioxidants, vitamins, minerals, and fiber. Enjoy every bite, knowing you're eating something that's good for you.

2 cups halved strawberries
2 cups cubed cantaloupe
2 cups cubed pineapple
2 kiwifruits, peeled and cubed
1 cup fat-free vanilla frozen yogurt, softened
½ teaspoon grated orange zest
⅛ teaspoon ground nutmeg
¼ cup dried cherries
¼ cup chopped macadamia nuts

1 In each of 8 dessert bowls place ¼ cup each strawberries, cantaloupe, and pineapple and 2 tablespoons kiwi.

2 In small bowl stir together frozen yogurt, zest, and nutmeg. Divide frozen yogurt mixture over fruit. Top each bowl with ½ tablespoon cherries and ½ tablespoon nuts.

Makes 8 servings

PER SERVING
116 calories / 3 g total fat / 23 calories from fat / 20% calories from fat
0 mg cholesterol / 24 mg sodium / 23 g carbohydrate / 3 g fiber / 17 g sugars / 3 g protein

moving forward
Keep the late-night munchies healthy with a low-fat snack such as fresh fruit, pretzels, or low-fat popcorn.

Lemon-Strawberry Sorbet

Prep Time: 5 minutes

You can enjoy the fresh flavors of strawberries year-round with this refreshing treat. For a change of pace, try using lime juice instead of lemon and add a pinch of ginger.

　　2　cups whole frozen strawberries
　　¼　cup lemon juice
　　2　tablespoons honey
　　2　cups plain low-fat yogurt

1 In blender process strawberries, lemon juice, and honey for 2 minutes or until shaved.

2 Add yogurt and blend just until mixture comes together, scraping down sides.

Makes 4 servings

PER SERVING
140 calories / 2 g total fat / 19 calories from fat / 14% calories from fat
7 mg cholesterol / 89 mg sodium / 25 g carbohydrate / 2 g fiber / 21 g sugars / 7 g protein

Blueberry Polka Dot Pops

Prep Time: 5 minutes ■ Freeze Time: 2 hours

These whimsical, easy-to-make pops are perfect for summer birthday parties, beach picnics, and days you need an in-a-hurry dessert.

　　2½　cups low-fat lemon yogurt
　　1　cup whipped cream (from pressurized can)
　　1½　cups blueberries

1 In small bowl gently stir together yogurt and whipped cream. Stir in blueberries.

2 Divide mixture among eight 5-ounce paper molds. Add 1 craft stick to each mold. Freeze for 2 hours or until set.

Makes 8 servings

PER SERVING
100 calories / 3 g total fat / 24 calories from fat / 24% calories from fat
10 mg cholesterol / 61 mg sodium / 15 g carbohydrate / 1 g fiber / 14 g sugars / 4 g protein

Red Velvet Cake

Prep Time: 10 minutes ■ Bake Time: 30 minutes

When preparing this cake, it may seem as though there's not enough batter for the pan because it only comes up ½ inch. But fear not: As the cake bakes it literally rises to the occasion. When baking in glass dishes—this cake or any other—always reduce the oven temperature by 25°F to prevent burning.

Cake

2¼	cups all-purpose flour
2	tablespoons unsweetened cocoa powder
1	teaspoon baking powder
1	teaspoon baking soda
1	teaspoon salt
1	cup fat-free (skim) milk
1	tablespoon distilled white vinegar
1	teaspoon vanilla
1	teaspoon liquid red food coloring
1½	cups granulated sugar
⅓	cup light olive oil
4	egg whites

Glaze

½	cup powdered sugar
2	tablespoons fat-free (skim) milk
½	teaspoon vanilla

1 Preheat oven to 350°F. Lightly spray 13×9-inch baking pan with nonstick cooking spray; dust with flour.

2 In medium bowl combine flour, cocoa powder, baking powder, baking soda, and salt. In another bowl combine milk, vinegar, vanilla, and food coloring.

3 In large mixing bowl beat granulated sugar and oil with electric mixer on medium speed until blended. Beat in egg whites, 1 at a time. Beat in flour mixture alternately with milk mixture, starting and ending with flour mixture. Spread batter in prepared pan.

4 Bake for 30 minutes or until wooden toothpick inserted in center of cake comes out clean. Place pan on wire rack to cool completely.

5 Meanwhile, prepare glaze. In small bowl whisk together powdered sugar, milk, and vanilla until smooth.

6 Drizzle glaze over cooled cake. To cut make 5 evenly spaced cuts on long side at 2¼-inch intervals and 3 evenly spaced cuts on short side at about 2⅜-inch intervals for total of 24 rectangular pieces. Cover and store in refrigerator for up to 3 days.

Makes 24 servings

PER SERVING
131 calories / 3 g total fat / 27 calories from fat / 21% calories from fat
0 mg cholesterol / 187 mg sodium / 24 g carbohydrate / 0 g fiber / 16 g sugars / 2 g protein

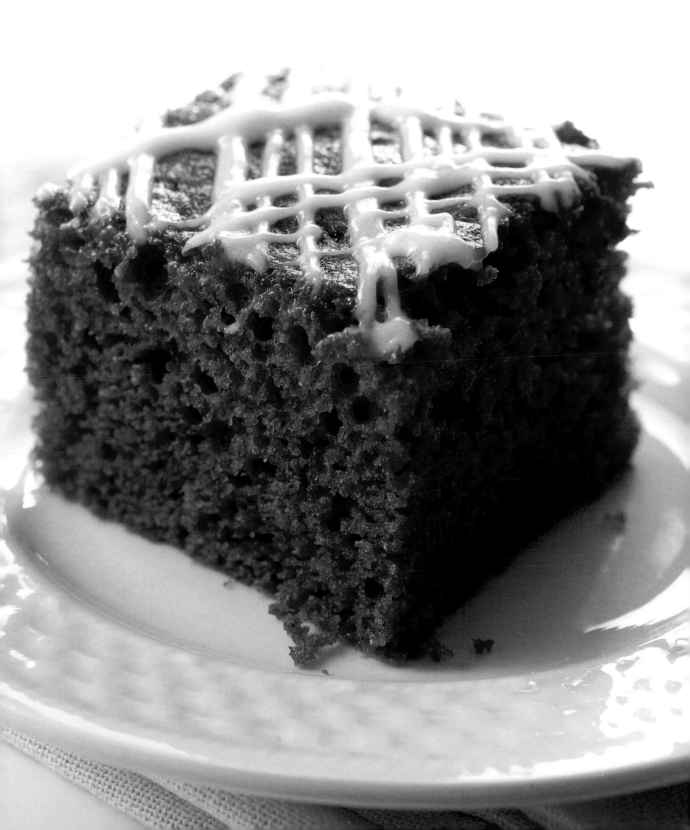

Flourless Chocolate-Almond Cake

Prep Time: 20 minutes ■ Bake Time: 35 minutes

This rich, dense cake highlights the classic chocolate and almond flavor combination. If you don't have almond extract, the cake is just as delicious without it.

4	tablespoons cocoa powder
¼	cup slivered almonds
¾	cup granulated sugar
3	ounces semisweet chocolate or chocolate pieces
1	tablespoon butter
1	6-ounce container fat-free chocolate yogurt
¼	teaspoon almond extract (optional)
8	egg whites
¼	teaspoon salt
1	tablespoon powdered sugar

1 Preheat oven to 350°F. Lightly spray 9-inch springform pan with nonstick cooking spray. Dust pan with 1 tablespoon of the cocoa powder.

2 In food processor combine almonds and 2 tablespoons of the granulated sugar. Process until finely ground.

3 In small saucepan melt chocolate and butter over low heat until smooth, stirring often. Or microwave at 15-second intervals, stirring after each.

4 In large bowl combine melted chocolate mixture, almond mixture, yogurt, almond extract (if desired), ½ cup of the remaining granulated sugar, and remaining 3 tablespoons cocoa powder.

5 In large mixing bowl beat egg whites and salt with electric mixer on high speed until foamy. Gradually beat in remaining 2 tablespoons granulated sugar until stiff peaks form. Gently fold in chocolate mixture until no streaks of egg white remain. Gently spread batter in prepared pan.

6 Bake for 35 minutes or until toothpick inserted in center of cake comes out with just a few moist crumbs clinging. Place on rack to cool slightly. (Cake will rise in oven, then shrink from sides of pan and fall as it cools.) Loosen edge of cake with knife or cake spatula and remove sides of pan. Cool completely.

7 To serve, place cake on serving plate and sprinkle with powdered sugar.

Makes 16 servings

PER SERVING
103 calories / 3 g total fat / 30 calories from fat / 29% calories from fat
2 mg cholesterol / 84 mg sodium / 17 g carbohydrate / 1 g fiber / 15 g sugars / 3 g protein

Banana Cake

Prep Time: 15 minutes ■ Bake Time: 35 minutes

This cake is very moist and will keep well for 5 days. To avoid the temptation of having cake around the house, cut it into individual pieces and freeze them in snack bags. Then for lunch boxes, last-minute company, or an occasional treat, thaw the cake pieces at room temperature.

	Nonstick cooking spray
1½	cups all-purpose flour
1	cup whole wheat pastry flour
1½	teaspoons baking soda
½	teaspoon salt
2	teaspoons ground cinnamon
½	teaspoon ground nutmeg
6	tablespoons butter, softened
1½	cups sugar
1¼	cups unsweetened applesauce
3	very ripe bananas, mashed
3	egg whites
1	teaspoon vanilla

1 Preheat oven to 350°F. Coat 13×9-inch baking pan with nonstick cooking spray.

2 In small bowl combine all-purpose flour, pastry flour, baking soda, salt, cinnamon, and nutmeg. Set aside.

3 In medium mixing bowl cream butter and sugar with electric mixer on medium speed until light and fluffy. Beat in applesauce, bananas, egg whites, and vanilla until smooth.

4 Add flour mixture to banana mixture and beat just until blended. Spread batter in prepared pan.

5 Bake for 35 minutes or until toothpick inserted in center comes out clean. Cool in pan for 10 minutes. Turn cake out onto wire rack to cool completely.

6 To cut cake make 4 evenly spaced cuts on long side at approximately 2½-inch intervals and 4 evenly spaced cuts on the short side at approximately 1½-inch intervals for a total of 25 rectangular pieces.

Makes 25 servings

PER SERVING
130 calories / 3 g total fat / 25 calories from fat / 19% calories from fat
7 mg cholesterol / 148 mg sodium / 25 g carbohydrate / 1 g fiber / 16 g sugars / 2 g protein

Lemon Angel Cake with Raspberry Syrup

Prep Time: 15 minutes

Starting with a store-bought cake makes this showstopping dessert ready in just minutes. A staple in England, lemon curd is with the jams and jellies in your supermarket or in the international section.

- 3 cups raspberries
- 2 tablespoons sugar
- 1 prepared angel food cake (9-inch)
- ½ cup lemon curd
- 1½ cups whipped cream (from pressurized can)

1 In medium bowl gently toss together raspberries and sugar. Set aside.

2 Cut cake into thirds horizontally. Place bottom layer of the cake on serving plate. Spread with half of the lemon curd and half of the whipped cream. Top with middle layer of the cake and repeat layers. Top with top layer of the cake. Cut into 12 slices and place on dessert plates. Divide raspberry syrup over slices.

Makes 12 servings

PER SERVING
152 calories / 3 g total fat / 24 calories from fat / 16% calories from fat
20 mg cholesterol / 231 mg sodium / 31 g carbohydrate / 0 g fiber / 18 g sugars / 3 g protein

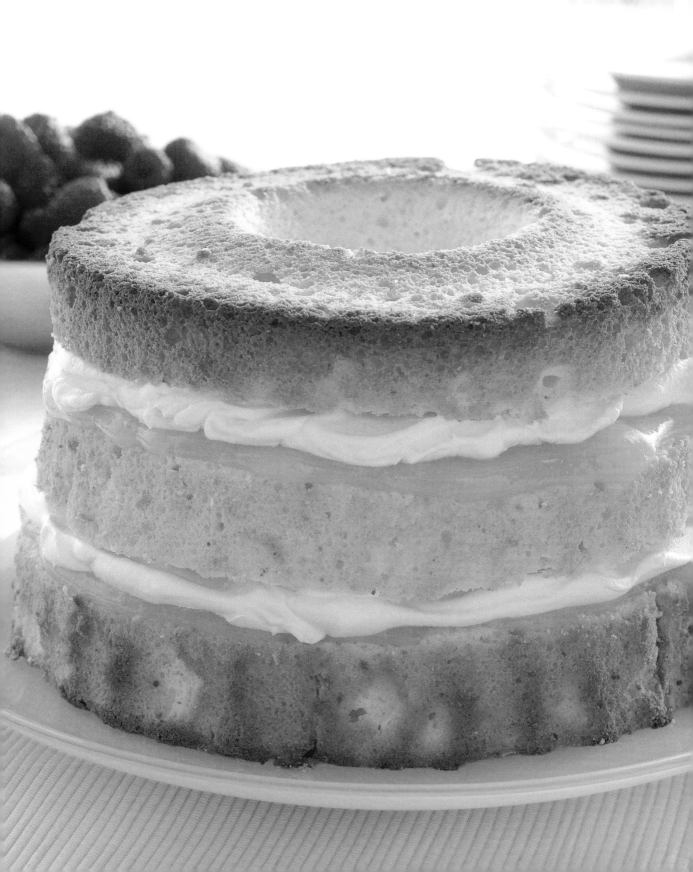

Peach-Raspberry Tart

Prep Time: 15 minutes ■ Bake Time: 15 minutes

Most pie or tart crusts are loaded with fat. This tender crust starts with oats to form a delicious base for flavorful fruit.

Crust		Filling	
	Nonstick cooking spray	5	small peaches
¾	cup rolled oats	2	tablespoons seedless raspberry all-fruit jam, melted
½	cup all-purpose flour		
¼	cup sugar	½	cup raspberries
¼	teaspoon salt		
3	tablespoons low-fat plain yogurt		
2	tablespoons light olive oil		

1 Preheat oven to 375°F. Line baking sheet with foil. Lightly spray foil with nonstick cooking spray.

2 In medium bowl combine oats, flour, sugar, and salt. Stir in yogurt and oil until soft dough forms.

3 Working on baking sheet, press or gently roll dough out with floured rolling pin to 10-inch circle. Pinch edge of circle slightly all around to form slight rim.

4 Bake crust for 15 minutes or until golden around edge. Place on wire rack to cool slightly.

5 Meanwhile, peel, halve, and thinly slice peaches.

6 Brush half of the jam over crust. Arrange peach slices in concentric circles on pastry. Brush with remaining jam. Scatter raspberries on top.

Makes 10 servings

PER SERVING
112 calories / 3 g total fat / 29 calories from fat / 26% calories from fat
0 mg cholesterol / 62 mg sodium / 19 g carbohydrate / 1 g fiber / 9 g sugars / 2 g protein

Crustless Pumpkin Pie

Prep Time: 5 minutes ■ Bake Time: 45 minutes

Most of the fat in pies comes from the crust. Here, without a crust, all that's left is healthful custardy goodness seasoned with warming spices and refreshing orange zest. Store the pie, covered, in the refrigerator for up to 5 days.

	Nonstick cooking spray
1	15-ounce can pumpkin puree
1¼	cups fat-free (skim) milk
2	eggs
2	tablespoons butter, melted
¾	cup sugar
1	tablespoon grated orange zest
½	teaspoon ground cinnamon
¼	teaspoon ground ginger
⅛	teaspoon ground nutmeg

1 Preheat oven to 350°F. Lightly spray 9-inch deep-dish pie plate with nonstick cooking spray.

2 In large bowl whisk together pumpkin, milk, eggs, butter, sugar, zest, cinnamon, ginger, and nutmeg. Pour into prepared pie plate.

3 Bake for 45 minutes or until knife inserted in center comes out clean. Place pie plate on wire rack to cool completely.

Makes 10 servings

PER SERVING
120 calories / 3 g total fat / 31 calories from fat / 26% calories from fat
49 mg cholesterol / 45 mg sodium / 20 g carbohydrate / 2 g fiber / 18 g sugars / 3 g protein

Apple-Cranberry Crumble

Prep Time: 15 minutes ■ Cook Time: 15 minutes

Fruit crumbles are a classic comfort food, especially when they're served warm. Refrigerate any remaining crumble and enjoy it cold as well.

Nonstick cooking spray
4 large sweet apples, peeled, halved, cored, and cut into ¼-inch slices
¼ cup dried sweetened cranberries
1 tablespoon water
1 tablespoon plus ¼ cup packed light brown sugar
3 tablespoons all-purpose flour
2 tablespoons rolled oats
2 tablespoons butter, cut up

1 Preheat oven to 450°F. Lightly spray 9-inch square baking pan with nonstick cooking spray.

2 In large saucepan combine apples, cranberries, the water, and 1 tablespoon of the brown sugar. Cook over medium-low heat, stirring occasionally, for 6 minutes or until apples begin to soften.

3 Meanwhile, in small bowl combine flour, oats, butter, and remaining ¼ cup brown sugar. Knead mixture with your fingers until well combined and crumbly.

4 Place hot apple mixture in prepared pan. Sprinkle evenly with crumb mixture.

5 Bake for 8 minutes or until crumb topping is firm and lightly brown.

Makes 9 servings

PER SERVING
118 calories / 3 g total fat / 23 calories from fat / 19% calories from fat
7 mg cholesterol / 20 mg sodium / 25 g carbohydrate / 4 g fiber / 18 g sugars / 0 g protein

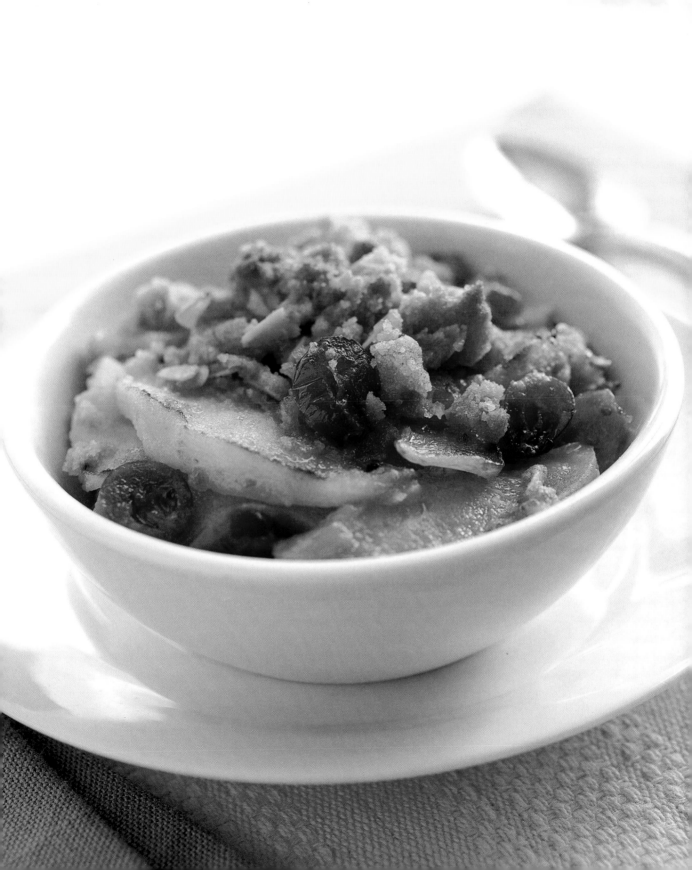

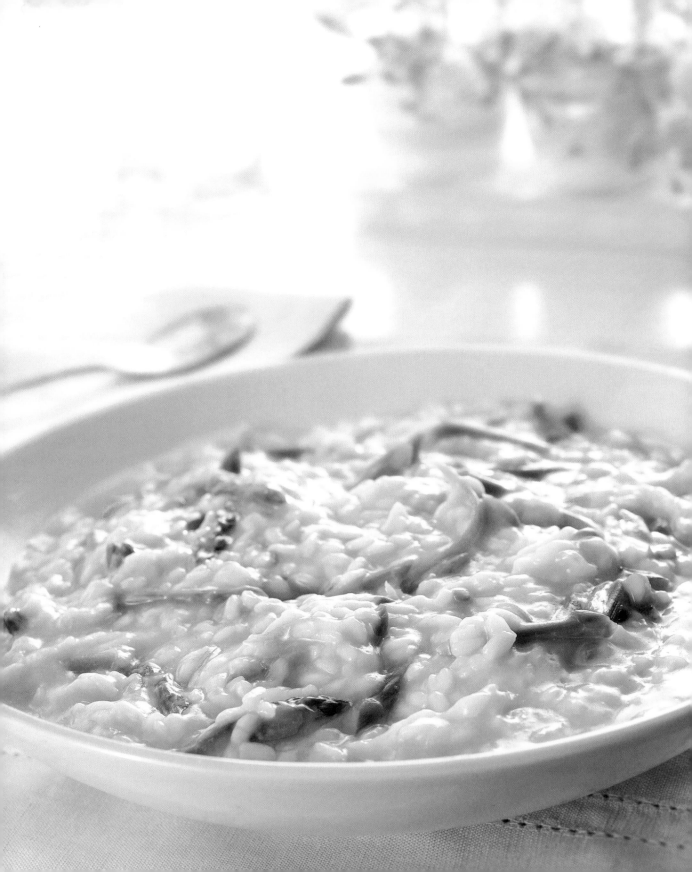

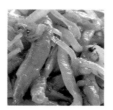

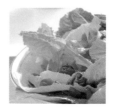

holidays

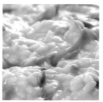

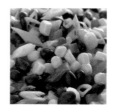

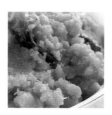

◀ Spring Asparagus Risotto, page 242

PASSOVER DINNER

Sweet Potato Tzimmes	238
Noodle Kugel	238
Honey-Glazed Green Beans	240

EASTER DINNER

Spring Asparagus Risotto	242
Baby Spinach Salad with Strawberries	244
Sweet Pea Soup with Pancetta	244

FOURTH OF JULY BARBECUE

Corn and Bean Salad	246
Potato Salad with Lemon Dressing	246
Zucchini and Carrot Slaw	248

THANKSGIVING DINNER

Green Beans with Caramelized Onions	250
Sweet Potato Casserole	250
Sausage-Vegetable Dressing	252

CHRISTMAS DINNER

Greens with Cranberry Vinaigrette	254
Scalloped Potatoes	256
Broccoli with Lemon and Red Pepper Flakes	257

PASSOVER DINNER

This springtime celebration features traditional favorites bursting with delicious, time-honored flavors. Gather family and friends because this hearty meal serves 12—or plan on leftovers later in the week. When preparing the Espresso Jelly, you'll want to triple the recipe because the original serves only 4.

PASSOVER DINNER

MAIN COURSE: Oven-Braised Beef Brisket (brisket recipe only) (page 128)
SIDE DISHES: Sweet Potato Tzimmes, Noodle Kugel, Honey-Glazed Green Beans
DESSERT: Espresso Jelly (triple recipe to serve 12) (page 210)

PASSOVER DINNER
Makes 12 servings
COMPLETE MEAL SERVING
515 calories / 9 g total fat / 88 calories from fat / 17% calories from fat
92 mg cholesterol / 594 mg sodium / 80 g carbohydrate / 8 g fiber / 45 g sugars / 27 g protein

OVEN-BRAISED BRISKET
Makes 12 servings
PER SERVING
148 calories / 5 g total fat / 46 calories from fat / 32% calories from fat
48 mg cholesterol / 142 mg sodium / 7 g carbohydrate / 0 g fiber / 7 g sugars / 17 g protein

SWEET POTATO TZIMMES
Makes 12 servings
PER SERVING
120 calories / 0 g total fat / 2 calories from fat / 0% calories from fat
0 mg cholesterol / 32 mg sodium / 29 g carbohydrate / 4 g fiber / 12 g sugars / 2 g protein

NOODLE KUGEL
Makes 24 servings
PER SERVING
84 calories / 1 g total fat / 11 calories from fat / 13% calories from fat
44 mg cholesterol / 152 mg sodium / 15 g carbohydrate / 1 g fiber / 4 g sugars / 3 g protein

HONEY-GLAZED GREEN BEANS
Makes 12 servings
PER SERVING
63 calories / 1 g total fat / 8 calories from fat / 12% calories from fat
0 mg cholesterol / 256 mg sodium / 13 g carbohydrate / 3 g fiber / 8 g sugars / 2 g protein

ESPRESSO JELLY (TRIPLE RECIPE TO SERVE 12)
Makes 4 servings
PER SERVING
100 calories / 2 g total fat / 21 calories from fat / 21% calories from fat
0 mg cholesterol / 12 mg sodium / 16 g carbohydrate / 0 g fiber / 14 g sugars / 3 g protein

Sweet Potato Tzimmes

Prep Time: 5 minutes ■ Cook Time: 50 minutes

3 pounds sweet potatoes, peeled and cut into ½-inch pieces
1 8-ounce can crushed pineapple, drained
⅓ cup dried plums (prunes), quartered
½ cup orange juice
2 tablespoons packed brown sugar
1 teaspoon ground cinnamon
½ teaspoon ground ginger

1 In large saucepan cook sweet potato in enough boiling water to cover for 10 minutes or until tender. Drain.

2 Preheat oven to 400°F. Lightly spray 2-quart baking dish with nonstick cooking spray.

3 In medium bowl coarsely mash sweet potato. Stir in pineapple, plums, orange juice, brown sugar, cinnamon, and ginger. Place in prepared baking dish. Cover and bake for 40 minutes or until heated through.

Makes 12 servings

For nutritional information see page 237

Noodle Kugel

Prep Time: 20 minutes ■ Cook Time: 1 hour

1 12-ounce bag whole wheat extra-wide noodles
5 large eggs
1 cup chicken broth
⅓ cup sugar
1 teaspoon salt
1 teaspoon vanilla
⅓ cup golden raisins

1 Cook noodles according to package directions. Drain, rinse with cold water, and drain well.

2 Preheat oven to 350°F. Lightly spray 13×9-inch baking dish with nonstick cooking spray; set aside.

3 In large bowl whisk together eggs, broth, sugar, salt, and vanilla. Add noodles and raisins and toss to coat. Place in prepared baking dish. Bake, uncovered, for 45 minutes or until knife inserted in center comes out clean.

Makes 24 servings

For nutritional information see page 237

Sweet Potato Tzimmes ▶

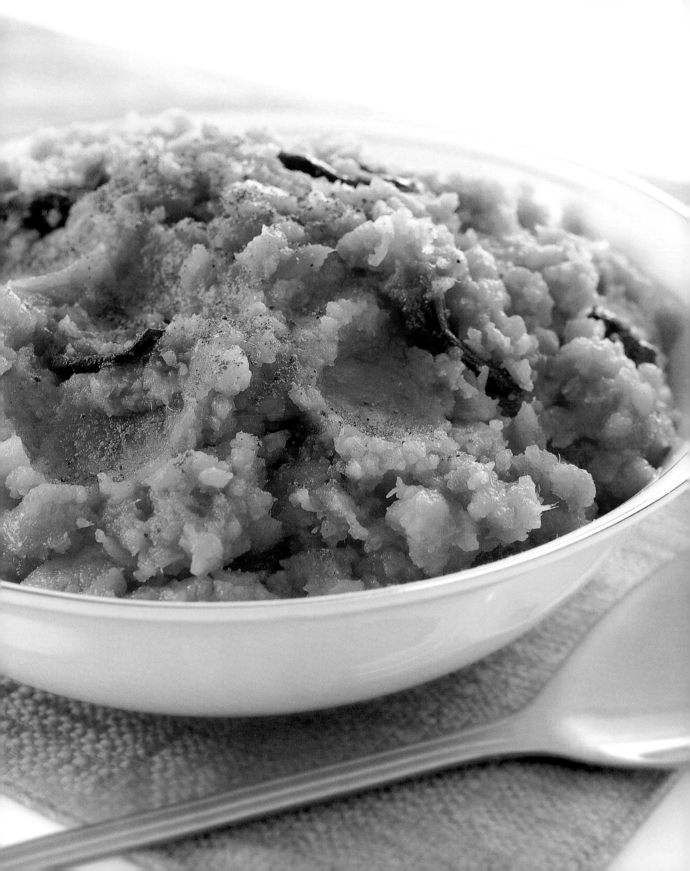

Honey-Glazed Green Beans

Prep Time: 10 minutes ■ Cook Time: 25 minutes

2	pounds green beans, trimmed
¼	teaspoon salt
⅛	teaspoon ground black pepper
1	teaspoon sesame oil
1	cup reduced-sodium chicken broth
½	cup orange juice
¼	cup honey
2	tablespoons soy sauce
1	tablespoon finely chopped fresh ginger
1	tablespoon sesame seeds, toasted

1 In large nonstick skillet cook green beans, salt, and pepper in hot oil over medium heat for 8 minutes or until lightly brown, stirring occasionally.

2 In medium bowl combine broth, orange juice, honey, soy sauce, and ginger. Add broth mixture to skillet. Bring to boiling; reduce heat to medium and cook, stirring occasionally, for 12 minutes or until beans are tender. With slotted spoon remove beans to serving bowl; keep warm.

3 Bring sauce to boiling and continue to boil for 5 minutes or until reduced by half. Pour sauce over beans and sprinkle with sesame seeds.

Makes 12 servings

For nutritional information see page 237

moving forward

Limit alcoholic drinks, which have too many empty calories and can affect your appetite.

EASTER DINNER

This Easter menu offers springtime favorites such as asparagus, peas, strawberries, and lamb. The meal feeds 10, except for the lamb and the cake, which serve 12. Be sure to measure out these dishes appropriately for the most accurate serving sizes. Happy Easter!

EASTER DINNER

APPETIZER: Sweet Pea Soup with Pancetta

MAIN COURSE: Grilled Boneless Leg of Lamb (lamb recipe only) (page 141)

SIDE DISH: Spring Asparagus Risotto

SALAD: Baby Spinach Salad with Strawberries

DESSERT: Lemon Angel Cake with Raspberry Syrup (page 228)

EASTER DINNER
Makes 10 servings
COMPLETE MEAL SERVING
616 calories / 14 g total fat / 118 calories from fat / 19% calories from fat
98 mg cholesterol / 1,518 mg sodium / 87 g carbohydrate / 9 g fiber / 32 g sugars / 41 g protein

SWEET PEA SOUP WITH PANCETTA
Makes 10 servings
PER SERVING
135 calories / 3 g total fat / 24 calories from fat / 18% calories from fat
11 mg cholesterol / 617 mg sodium / 19 g carbohydrate / 6 g fiber / 8 g sugars / 10 g protein

GRILLED BONELESS LEG OF LAMB
Makes 12 servings
PER SERVING
145 calories / 6 g total fat / 51 calories from fat / 37% calories from fat
65 mg cholesterol / 244 mg sodium / 1 g carbohydrate / 0 g fiber / 0 g sugars / 21 g protein

SPRING ASPARAGUS RISOTTO
Makes 10 servings
PER SERVING
155 calories / 2 g total fat / 17 calories from fat / 10% calories from fat
2 mg cholesterol / 322 mg sodium / 29 g carbohydrate / 1 g fiber / 3 g sugars / 6 g protein

BABY SPINACH SALAD WITH STRAWBERRIES
Makes 10 servings
PER SERVING
29 calories / 0 g total fat / 2 calories from fat / 0% calories from fat
0 mg cholesterol / 104 mg sodium / 7 g carbohydrate / 2 g fiber / 3 g sugars / 1 g protein

LEMON ANGEL CAKE WITH RASPBERRY SYRUP
Makes 12 servings
PER SERVING
152 calories / 3 g total fat / 24 calories from fat / 16% calories from fat
20 mg cholesterol / 231 mg sodium / 31 g carbohydrate / 0 g fiber / 18 g sugars / 3 g protein

Spring Asparagus Risotto

Prep Time: 5 minutes ■ Cook Time: 26 minutes

4½	cups fat-free, reduced-sodium chicken broth
1	cup chopped onion (1 large)
1	teaspoon olive oil
1	tablespoon water
1½	cups uncooked Arborio rice
¼	cup dry white wine
1	pound thin asparagus, trimmed and bias-sliced into 1-inch pieces
⅓	cup shredded carrot
2	tablespoons snipped fresh chives
¼	cup grated Parmesan cheese (1 ounce)

1 In medium saucepan, bring broth to simmering over high heat. Cover and remove from heat.

2 Meanwhile, in large saucepan cook and stir onion in hot oil and water over medium-high heat for 4 minutes or until softened. Add rice, stirring to coat with oil. Stir in wine and cook for 30 seconds or until completely evaporated. Stir in 3 cups of the warm broth. Bring to boiling, stirring constantly.

3 Reduce heat to low; cover and simmer for 10 minutes or until liquid is absorbed. Stir in remaining broth, asparagus, carrot, and chives. Bring mixture to boiling and cook for 1 minute, stirring constantly. Reduce heat to low; cover and simmer for 10 minutes or until rice and vegetables are tender and liquid is absorbed. Stir in cheese.

Makes 10 servings

For nutritional information see page 241

moving forward

Know when to say no. When your hostess tries to heap food on your plate, thank her kindly but refuse the extra.

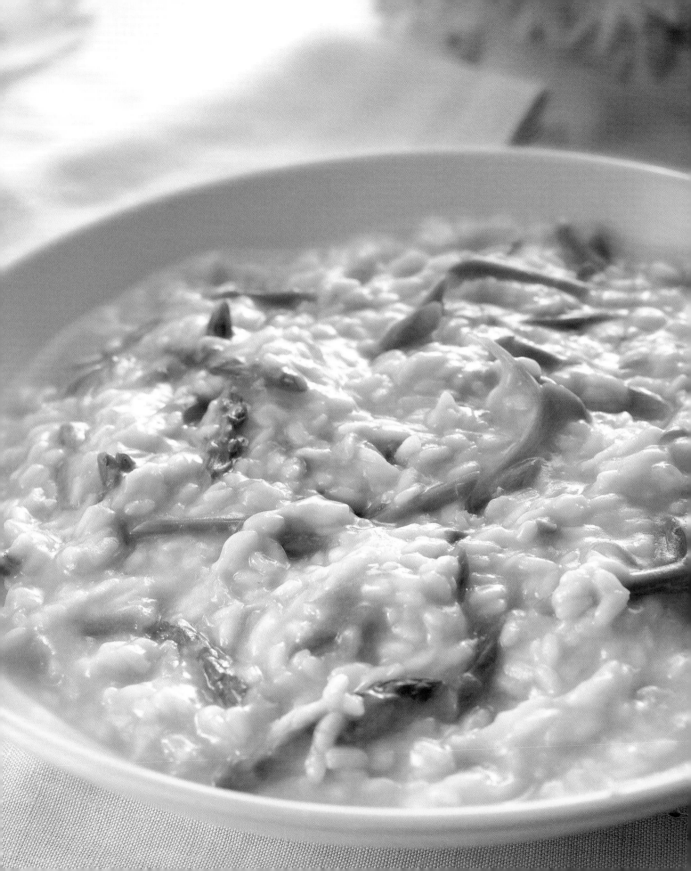

Baby Spinach Salad with Strawberries

Prep Time: 10 minutes

    4   cups strawberries, hulled and sliced
    ¼   cup fat-free red wine vinaigrette
    4   cups packed baby spinach leaves
    2   cups packed baby arugula
    1   cup endive, cut crosswise into ½-inch slices

1 Place half of the strawberries in blender or food processor; blend until smooth. Pour strawberry puree into small bowl. Whisk in vinaigrette.

2 In large serving bowl combine remaining strawberries, spinach, arugula, and endive. Add dressing and toss to coat.

Makes 10 servings

For nutritional information see page 241

Sweet Pea Soup with Pancetta

Prep Time: 5 minutes   ■   Cook Time: 20 minutes

    4   ounces pancetta, diced (⅔ cup)
    2   cups chopped onion (2 large)
    2   16-ounce packages frozen petite peas, thawed
    7   cups fat-free, reduced-sodium chicken broth
    1   cup reduced-fat (2%) milk
    3   tablespoons snipped fresh mint
    ⅓   cup reduced-fat sour cream

1 In large saucepan cook and stir pancetta over medium heat for 5 minutes or until crisp. With slotted spoon, remove pancetta to paper towels to drain.

2 Add onion to saucepan with drippings; cook and stir for 5 minutes. Add peas and broth. Increase heat to high; bring to boiling.

3 Reduce heat to low; cover and simmer for 10 minutes or until peas are very tender. Working in batches, place in food processor. Process until smooth. Return pea mixture to pan. Stir in milk and mint; heat through. Garnish each bowl with about ½ tablespoon sour cream.

Makes 10 servings

For nutritional information see page 241

FOURTH OF JULY BARBECUE

Gather your family and friends and light up the grill. Fourth of July is a holiday for outdoor fun—parades, pool parties, family gatherings, and picnics. This menu is high on flavor but short on work time. If you prefer, the salads can be made a day ahead, covered, and refrigerated until needed. If you're pulling together a last-minute bash, these come together in no time. Either way, it's a day for relaxing and enjoying yourself.

FOURTH OF JULY BARBECUE

MAIN COURSE: Grilled Flank Steak (steak recipe only) (page 124)
SALADS: Potato Salad with Lemon Dressing, Zucchini and Carrot Slaw, Corn and Bean Salad
DESSERT: Blueberry Polka Dot Pops (page 223)

FOURTH OF JULY BARBECUE

Makes 8 servings
COMPLETE MEAL SERVING
580 calories / 17 g total fat / 152 calories from fat / 26% calories from fat
81 mg cholesterol / 1,032 mg sodium / 68 g carbohydrate / 8 g fiber / 33 g sugars / 39 g protein

GRILLED FLANK STEAK

Makes 8 servings
PER SERVING
262 calories / 11 g total fat / 99 calories from fat / 38% calories from fat
68 mg cholesterol / 291 mg sodium / 11 g carbohydrate / 0 g fiber / 9 g sugars / 28 g protein

POTATO SALAD WITH LEMON DRESSING

Makes 8 servings
PER SERVING
100 calories / 0 g total fat / 4 calories from fat / 4% calories from fat
1 mg cholesterol / 163 mg sodium / 21 g carbohydrate / 2 g fiber / 3 g sugars / 3 g protein

ZUCCHINI AND CARROT SLAW

Makes 8 servings
PER SERVING
47 calories / 2 g total fat / 14 calories from fat / 30% calories from fat
2 mg cholesterol / 146 mg sodium / 8 g carbohydrate / 2 g fiber / 5 g sugars / 1 g protein

CORN AND BEAN SALAD

Makes 8 servings
PER SERVING
71 calories / 1 g total fat / 11 calories from fat / 15% calories from fat
0 mg cholesterol / 371 mg sodium / 13 g carbohydrate / 3 g fiber / 2 g sugars / 3 g protein

BLUEBERRY POLKA DOT POPS

Makes 8 servings
PER SERVING
100 calories / 3 g total fat / 24 calories from fat / 24% calories from fat
10 mg cholesterol / 61 mg sodium / 15 g carbohydrate / 1 g fiber / 14 g sugars / 4 g protein

Corn and Bean Salad

Prep Time: 15 minutes

- 1   clove garlic, crushed
- 1   teaspoon olive oil
- 1   tablespoon white wine vinegar or distilled white vinegar
- ½   teaspoon salt
- 1   15-ounce can black beans, rinsed and drained
- 1   15¼-ounce can whole kernel corn, drained
- 1   cup chopped red sweet pepper
- ½   cup chopped green onion (4)

1 Rub bottom of large salad bowl with garlic. Add oil, vinegar, and salt to bowl; whisk to blend.

2 Add beans, corn, sweet pepper, and green onion. Toss to coat well.

Makes 8 servings

For nutritional information see page 245

Potato Salad with Lemon Dressing

Prep Time: 15 minutes ■ Cook Time: 20 minutes

- 2   pounds red potatoes (6 medium), cut into ¾-inch chunks
- ½   cup plain low-fat yogurt
- 1   clove garlic, crushed
- 2   tablespoons lemon juice
- 1   tablespoon snipped fresh dill weed
- 1   teaspoon sugar
- ½   teaspoon lemon zest
- ½   teaspoon salt
- ½   cup chopped red onion

1 In large saucepan cook potato, covered, in enough boiling water to cover for 20 minutes or until tender. Drain, rinsing with cold water until cool.

2 Meanwhile, in large bowl whisk together yogurt, garlic, lemon juice, dill weed, sugar, zest, and salt. Add cooled potato and onion, tossing to coat well.

Makes 8 servings

For nutritional information see page 245

Corn and Bean Salad ▶

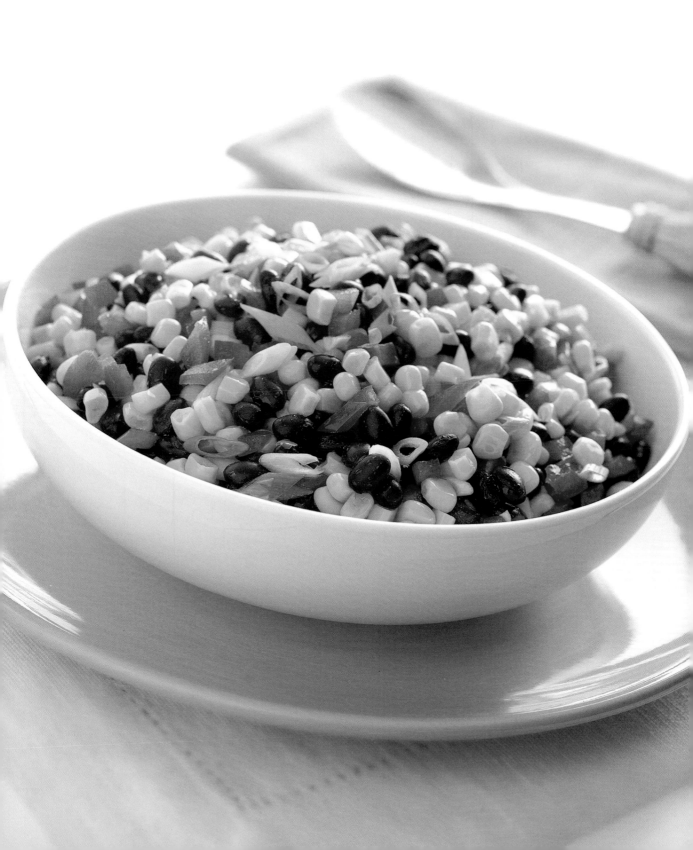

Zucchini and Carrot Slaw

Prep Time: 15 minutes

3	tablespoons low-fat mayonnaise
3	tablespoons reduced-fat sour cream
1	tablespoon apple cider vinegar
1	tablespoon lemon juice
1	teaspoon sugar
½	teaspoon celery seeds
¼	teaspoon salt
8	ounces zucchini, cut into julienne sticks (2½ cups)
8	ounces carrots, cut into julienne sticks (2½ cups)
1	apple, cut into matchsticks

In large bowl whisk together mayonnaise, sour cream, vinegar, lemon juice, sugar, celery seeds, and salt until blended. Stir in zucchini, carrot, and apple and toss to coat.

Makes 8 servings

For nutritional information see page 245

moving forward

Don't stand near the buffet at parties—if food is out of sight it may be out of mind.

THANKSGIVING DINNER

Celebrating a national holiday that focuses on food can certainly be challenging. No worries here; it's all figured out for you with classic recipes highlighting the favorite flavors of the season. Use your own turkey recipe. This meal is based on a 3-ounce serving of turkey breast, about the size and thickness of a deck of cards. Not only are these recipes delicious, they're also quick and easy. So relax, watch a parade or football game, and have a great day. Happy Thanksgiving!

THANKSGIVING DINNER

MAIN COURSE: 3 ounces skinless white turkey breast from your favorite roast turkey
SIDE DISHES: Sweet Potato Casserole, Green Beans with Caramelized Onions, Sausage-Vegetable Dressing
DESSERT: Crustless Pumpkin Pie (page 231)

THANKSGIVING DINNER
Makes 8 servings
COMPLETE MEAL SERVING
507 calories / 9 g total fat / 82 calories from fat / 16% calories from fat
123 mg cholesterol / 883 mg sodium / 71 g carbohydrate / 10 g fiber / 37 g sugars / 38 g protein

ROASTED TURKEY BREAST (3-OUNCE SERVING)
Makes 8 servings
PER SERVING
115 calories / 1 g total fat / 6 calories from fat / 8% calories from fat
71 mg cholesterol / 44 mg sodium / 0 g carbohydrate / 0 g fiber / 0 g sugars / 26 g protein

SWEET POTATO CASSEROLE
Makes 8 servings
PER SERVING
115 calories / 3 g total fat / 25 calories from fat / 21% calories from fat
0 mg cholesterol / 152 mg sodium / 22 g carbohydrate / 2 g fiber / 14 g sugars / 1 g protein

GREEN BEANS WITH CARAMELIZED ONIONS
Makes 8 servings
PER SERVING
39 calories / 0 g total fat / 3 calories from fat / 6% calories from fat
0 mg cholesterol / 149 mg sodium / 9 g carbohydrate / 3 g fiber / 3 g sugars / 2 g protein

SAUSAGE-VEGETABLE DRESSING
Makes 8 servings
PER SERVING
118 calories / 2 g total fat / 17 calories from fat / 14% calories from fat
3 mg cholesterol / 493 mg sodium / 20 g carbohydrate / 3 g fiber / 2 g sugars / 6 g protein

CRUSTLESS PUMPKIN PIE
Makes 10 servings
PER SERVING
120 calories / 3 g total fat / 31 calories from fat / 26% calories from fat
49 mg cholesterol / 45 mg sodium / 20 g carbohydrate / 2 g fiber / 18 g sugars / 3 g protein

Green Beans with Caramelized Onions

Prep Time: 10 minutes ■ Cook Time: 25 minutes

1	teaspoon dried thyme, crushed
½	teaspoon salt
½	teaspoon sugar
2	medium onions, halved lengthwise and cut into ¼-inch slices
¼	cup water (optional)
1½	pounds green beans, trimmed

1 In medium saucepan lightly sprayed with nonstick cooking spray cook thyme, salt, sugar, and onion over medium-high heat for 15 minutes, stirring occasionally. Reduce heat to medium-low; cover and cook and stir for 10 minutes or until onion is soft and brown. If pan dries out, add the water.

2 Meanwhile, in medium saucepan cook beans, covered, in small amount of boiling water for 10 minutes or until crisp-tender; drain. Place beans in serving bowl and top with onions.

Makes 8 servings

For nutritional information see page 249

Sweet Potato Casserole

Prep Time: 10 minutes ■ Bake Time: 1 hour 40 minutes

1½	pounds sweet potatoes
½	cup apple juice
¼	cup maple syrup
2	tablespoons unsweetened applesauce
1	teaspoon ground cinnamon
½	teaspoon salt
¼	cup chopped pecans

1 Preheat oven to 375°F. Place potatoes on baking sheet and bake for 1 hour or until very tender. Remove and let cool slightly.

2 Lightly spray 2-quart baking dish with nonstick cooking spray. Cut each potato in half and scoop pulp into large mixing bowl. Beat potato with apple juice, maple syrup, applesauce, cinnamon, and salt with electric mixer on medium speed until smooth and blended. Spoon into prepared baking dish and top with pecans.

3 Cover and bake for 30 minutes. Uncover and bake for 10 minutes or until heated through.

Makes 8 servings

For nutritional information see page 249

Green Beans with Caramelized Onions ▶

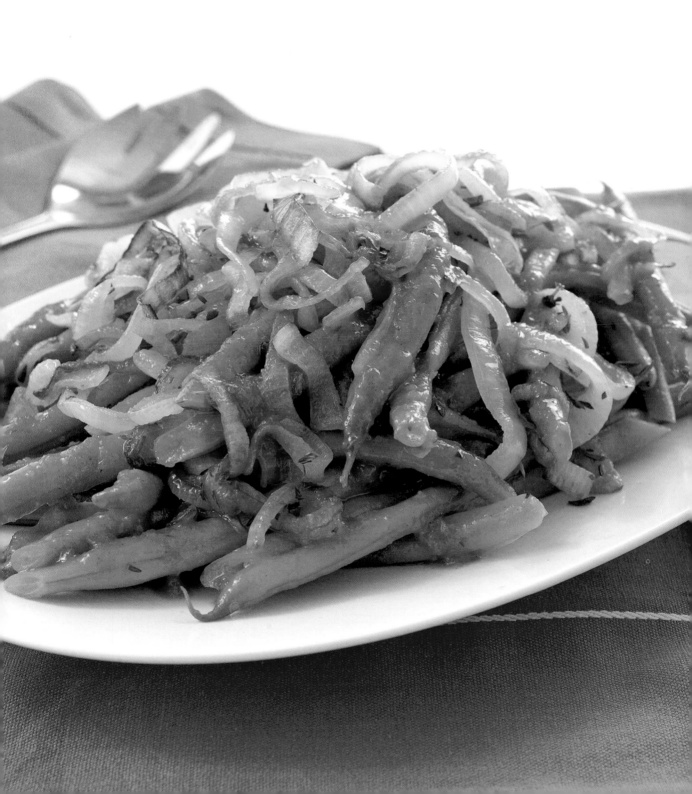

Sausage-Vegetable Dressing

Prep Time: 5 minutes ■ Cook Time: 40 minutes

    Nonstick cooking spray

4 ounces sweet turkey sausage, casings removed

1 teaspoon ground sage or poultry seasoning

1 16-ounce bag frozen assorted vegetables

1 teaspoon olive oil

6 ounces white soft bread cubes (about 5 cups)

2 14-ounce cans fat-free, reduced-sodium chicken broth

1 Preheat oven to 350°F. Lightly spray 2-quart baking dish with nonstick cooking spray.

2 In large nonstick skillet lightly sprayed with nonstick cooking spray cook and stir sausage and sage over medium-high heat for 5 minutes or until no longer pink. Drain any drippings. Place in prepared baking dish.

3 Add vegetables to skillet and cook and stir in hot oil for 5 minutes or until vegetables are lightly browned and heated through. Remove from heat; stir in bread cubes and broth; toss gently until moistened. Place in prepared baking dish and toss to coat.

4 Cover and bake for 30 minutes or until heated through.

Makes 8 servings

For nutritional information see page 249

moving forward

When hosting a party, encourage each guest to take home a plate of leftovers. Then your fridge won't be left full of tasty temptations.

CHRISTMAS DINNER

You've decked the halls, hung the stockings, and wrapped the gifts. Now relax and relish the holiday. This simple, elegant Christmas dinner will impress your guests with little work on your end. Enjoy these delicious dishes with your favorite baked (extra-lean) ham, each serving the size and height of a deck of cards.

CHRISTMAS DINNER

MAIN COURSE: Baked extra-lean (5% fat) ham (3-ounce serving)

SIDE DISHES: Scalloped Potatoes, Broccoli with Lemon and Red Pepper Flakes

SALAD: Greens with Cranberry Vinaigrette

DESSERT: Flourless Chocolate-Almond Cake (page 226)

CHRISTMAS DINNER
Makes 8 servings
TO COMPLETE THE MEAL—Per serving: one 1-ounce whole wheat dinner roll (2½-inch)
COMPLETE MEAL SERVING
544 calories / 17 g total fat / 154 calories from fat / 28% calories from fat
54 mg cholesterol / 1,905 mg sodium / 69 g carbohydrate / 12 g fiber / 32 g sugars / 35 g protein

BAKED EXTRA-LEAN (5% FAT) HAM (3-OUNCE SERVING)
Makes 8 servings
PER SERVING
123 calories / 5 g total fat / 42 calories from fat / 34% calories from fat
45 mg cholesterol / 1,023 mg sodium / 1 g carbohydrate / 0 g fiber / 0 g sugars / 18 g protein

SCALLOPED POTATOES
Makes 8 servings
PER SERVING
102 calories / 2 g total fat / 22 calories from fat / 22% calories from fat
7 mg cholesterol / 343 mg sodium / 14 g carbohydrate / 4 g fiber / 5 g sugars / 5 g protein

BROCCOLI WITH LEMON AND RED PEPPER FLAKES
Makes 8 servings
PER SERVING
47 calories / 1 g total fat / 13 calories from fat / 28% calories from fat
1 mg cholesterol / 197 mg sodium / 7 g carbohydrate / 3 g fiber / 1 g sugars / 3 g protein

GREENS WITH CRANBERRY VINAIGRETTE
Makes 8 servings
PER SERVING
73 calories / 4 g total fat / 31 calories from fat / 39% calories from fat
0 mg cholesterol / 86 mg sodium / 11 g carbohydrate / 2 g fiber / 8 g sugars / 2 g protein

FLOURLESS CHOCOLATE-ALMOND CAKE
Makes 16 servings
PER SERVING
103 calories / 3 g total fat / 30 calories from fat / 29% calories from fat
2 mg cholesterol / 84 mg sodium / 17 g carbohydrate / 1 g fiber / 15 g sugars / 3 g protein

Greens with Cranberry Vinaigrette

Prep Time: 10 minutes

½   cup cranberry juice

⅓   cup chopped fresh cranberries

½   tablespoon plus ½ teaspoon apple cider vinegar

½   teaspoon Dijon mustard

¼   teaspoon salt

¼   teaspoon sugar

1   teaspoon olive oil

6   cups torn romaine lettuce

2   cups packed arugula leaves

2   oranges, rind and pith removed, cut lengthwise in half, then sliced (2 cups)

¼   cup pecans, toasted

1 In large bowl whisk together cranberry juice, cranberries, vinegar, mustard, salt, and sugar. Whisk in oil.

2 Add lettuce, arugula, orange slices, and pecans and toss to coat well.

Makes 8 servings

For nutritional information see page 253

moving forward

Eat before you meet. Have a pre-party snack, such as an apple or low-fat popcorn, so you won't be tempted to nosh on high-calorie, high-fat party foods.

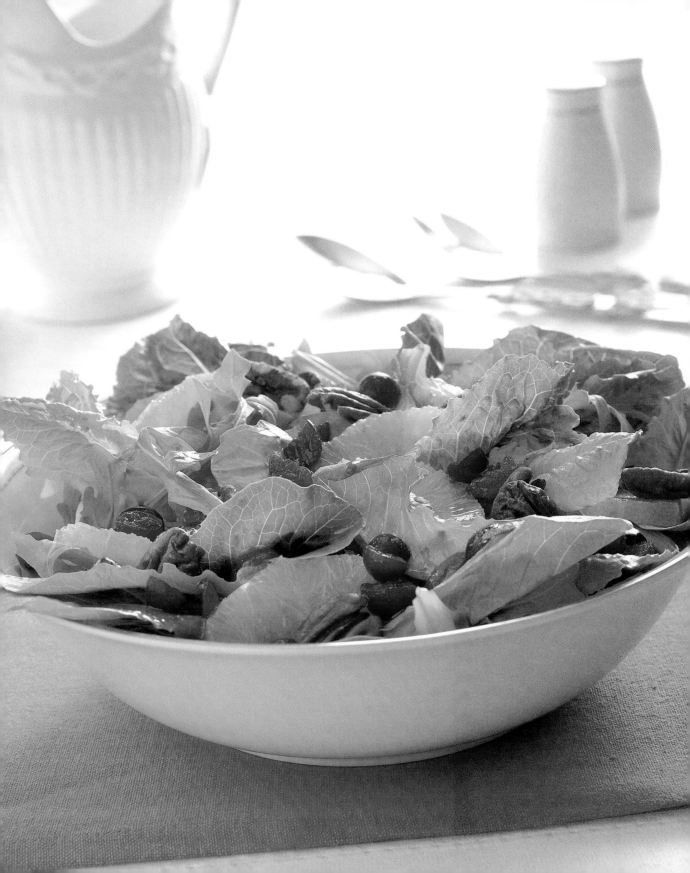

Scalloped Potatoes

Prep Time: 15 minutes ■ Cook Time: 1 hour 5 minutes

Nonstick cooking spray
1 cup sliced onion (1)
2 large cloves garlic, minced
½ cup sliced green onion (4)
1 10¾-ounce can condensed 98% fat-free cream of mushroom soup
1¼ cups reduced-fat (2%) milk
¼ cup shredded Parmesan cheese (1 ounce)
2 pounds baking potatoes, scrubbed and cut into ¼-inch slices
2 tablespoons all-purpose flour
¼ teaspoon ground black pepper

1 Preheat oven to 400°F. Lightly spray 8-inch square baking dish with nonstick cooking spray.

2 In large nonstick skillet lightly sprayed with nonstick cooking spray cook onion, garlic, and green onion over medium heat for 5 minutes, stirring occasionally.

3 Meanwhile, in medium saucepan whisk together soup and milk. Bring to simmer over medium-high heat. Remove from heat and stir in cheese.

4 While soup comes to simmer, arrange half of the potato slices in single layer, overlapping slightly, on bottom of prepared baking dish. Sprinkle with 1 tablespoon of the flour and ⅛ teaspoon of the pepper. Spread onion mixture on top of potato. Repeat layering with remaining potato, flour, and pepper.

5 Carefully pour soup mixture over potato slices. Cover and bake for 40 minutes. Uncover and bake for 20 minutes or until potato is tender. Remove from oven and let stand 5 minutes before serving.

Makes 8 servings

For nutritional information see page 253

Broccoli with Lemon and Red Pepper Flakes

Prep Time: 10 minutes ■ Cook Time: 15 minutes

8	cups broccoli florets
	Nonstick cooking spray
2	tablespoons plain dry bread crumbs
1	tablespoon pine nuts, coarsely chopped
2	large cloves garlic, sliced
½	teaspoon crushed red pepper flakes
1	cup chopped red sweet pepper (1)
1	teaspoon grated lemon zest
½	teaspoon salt
2	tablespoons grated Parmesan cheese

1 In large saucepan cook broccoli, covered, in small amount of boiling water for 6 minutes or until crisp-tender. Drain well.

2 Meanwhile, in large nonstick skillet lightly sprayed with nonstick cooking spray cook bread crumbs and nuts over medium heat for 2 minutes or until toasted. Remove to bowl; set aside.

3 Wipe skillet clean. In same skillet coated with nonstick cooking spray cook garlic and red pepper flakes over medium heat for 1 minute or until lightly brown. Add sweet pepper and cook and stir for 4 minutes or until tender. Add broccoli, zest, and salt; cook and stir for 1 minute or until heated through.

4 Place broccoli mixture in serving bowl. Sprinkle with bread crumb mixture and cheese.

Makes 8 servings
For nutritional information see page 253

easy alli® meal plans

The twenty-one menus here are designed around the recipes in this book to give you an idea on how to organize your daily meal plans. You'll find three weeks of menus including breakfast, lunch, dinner, and two snacks for each of the 1,200, 1,400, 1,600, and 1,800 calorie targets. If a recipe title is listed in a meal plan, it refers to the recipe itself. If a recipe is listed with the word "breakfast," "lunch," or "dinner" following it, it refers to the recipe and the side accompaniments that are listed in the "To Complete the Meal" portion of the recipe page.

The meal plans are alli-friendly--all calculated to contain the correct amount of calories and fat and to evenly distribute fat intake throughout the day so you consume no more than 30 percent calories from fat at each meal. When you are planning meals on your own, you should try to achieve the following targets:

	1,200 calories	1,400 calories	1,600 calories	1,800 calories
Fat grams per meal	12 grams	15 grams	17 grams	19 grams
Daily fat gram total	39 grams	48 grams	54 grams	60 grams

These meals plans were also designed to be balanced and healthy. Here are some helpful tips to keep in mind for healthy meal planning.

- Have no more than 10 percent calories from saturated fat daily.

- Keep your cholesterol at about 300 milligrams per day.

- Keep your sodium intake below 2,300 milligrams per day.

- Have two servings of fish per week.

- Limit trans fats as much as possible.

To keep within your calorie and fat targets, these meal plans should be followed in their entirety, however, if there is a meal that doesn't suit your taste or your schedule, you can substitute with another meal that has the same (or as close to the same as possible) calories and fat grams.

Now all you have to do is take a look through these easy alli meal plans, choose your favorite, and enjoy!

Week 1 Day 1

	1,200 CALORIES	1,400 CALORIES	1,600 CALORIES	1,800 CALORIES
BREAKFAST	Broccoli Cheese Omelet Breakfast (p.26); 6 oz. reduced-fat (2%) milk	Broccoli Cheese Omelet Breakfast (p.26); 6 oz. reduced-fat (2%) milk; 1 small orange	Broccoli Cheese Omelet Breakfast (p.26) w/ 2 T. ⅓ less-fat cream cheese; 1 ½ c. honeydew melon balls	Broccoli Cheese Omelet Breakfast (p.26) w/ 2 T. light cream cheese; 1 c. honeydew mellon balls; 6 almonds
LUNCH	Quinoa, Veggie, and Pork Toss (p.53)	Quinoa, Veggie, and Pork Toss (p.53); ½ medium apple; 5 large green olives	Quinoa, Veggie, and Pork Toss (p.53); 4 large black olives; ½ c. canned peaches	Quinoa, Veggie, and Pork Toss (p.53); 3 dried figs; 4 walnuts; 3 black olives
SNACK	1 small orange	Trail Mix (p.190)	Trail Mix (p.190); 1 small orange	Trail Mix (p.190); 1 small orange
DINNER	Tex-Mex Mini Meat Loaves Dinner (p.105)	Tex-Mex Mini Meat Loaves Dinner (p.105) w/ 1 T. avocado	Tex-Mex Mini Meat Loaves Dinner (p.105) w/ 1 ½ T. avocado; 2 T. non-fat sour cream	Tex-Mex Mini Meat Loaves Dinner (p.105); 3 T. avocado; 1 medium banana
SNACK	½ c. grapes	½ c. sugar-free flavored gelatin 4 T. light non-dairy whipped topping; ½ c. grapes	½ c. grapes w/ 6 T. light non-dairy whipped topping	½ c. sugar-free gelatin; ½ oz. light cheddar cheese
	38 grams fat / 1,239 calories	47.5 grams fat / 1,459 calories	53 grams fat / 1,625 calories	60.5 grams fat / 1,813 calories

Week 1 Day 2

	1,200 CALORIES	1,400 CALORIES	1,600 CALORIES	1,800 CALORIES
BREAKFAST	Fruit and Nut Granola Breakfast (p.8)	Fruit and Nut Granola Breakfast (p.8); 4 oz. reduced-fat (2%) milk	Fruit and Nut Granola Breakfast (p.8); 1 oz. light cheddar cheese; 2 fat-free crackers	Fruit and Nut Granola Breakfast (p.8); 1½ oz. light cheddar cheese; 1 medium orange
LUNCH	Roasted Vegetable Wrap (p.74)	Roasted Vegetable Wrap (p.74)	Roasted Vegetable Wrap (p.74)	Roasted Vegetable Wrap (p.74); Garbanzo Nuts (p.188); ½ c. peaches; ¼ c. light cottage cheese
SNACK	1/8 cantaloupe	16 oz. no calorie beverage	16 oz. no calorie beverage; 1 small banana	16 oz. no-calorie beverage; 6 dried apricot halves
DINNER	Rosemary Pork Roast Dinner (p.110)	Rosemary Pork Roast Dinner (p.110); Pears with Maple Crème (p.216)	Rosemary Pork Roast Dinner (p.110); Pears with Maple Crème (p.216); 2 T. light non-dairy whipped topping	Rosemary Pork Roast Dinner (p.110); Pears with Maple Crème (p.216); 6 raw almonds
SNACK	¼ c. salsa w/ ½ c. cucumber or jicama sticks	1 c. cucumber or jicama sticks; 2 tsp. light Ranch dressing	½ c. fat-free salsa w/ 2 T. light sour cream and 1 c. cucumber or jicama sticks	¼ c. fat-free salsa; 2 T. light cream cheese; ½ c. cucumber or jicama sticks
	39 grams fat / 1,250 calories	44.5 grams fat / 1,431 calories	51 grams fat / 1,616 calories	59 grams fat / 1,832 calories

Week 1 Day 3

	1,200 CALORIES	1,400 CALORIES	1,600 CALORIES	1,800 CALORIES
BREAKFAST	Peach-Almond Oatmeal Breakfast (p.6)	Peach-Almond Oatmeal Breakfast (p.6); 1 c. low-fat (1%) milk	Peach-Almond Oatmeal Breakfast (p.6); ½ medium banana; 1 c. reduced-fat (2%) milk	Peach-Almond Oatmeal Breakfast (p.6); 1 slice low-cal bread w/1 T. light spread; ½ medium banana; ½ oz. light cheddar cheese
LUNCH	Sensational Salmon Salad Lunch (p. 58)	Sensational Salmon Salad Lunch (p.58) 5 green olives; ½ c. fruit cocktail	Sensational Salmon Salad Lunch (p.58); 2 T. avocado; ½ pear	Sensational Salmon Salad Lunch (p.58); Buffalo-Style Crackers (p.190); 2 T. avocado; ¾ c. fruit cocktail
SNACK	Creamy Fruit Cup Snack (p.195)	Creamy Fruit Cup Snack (p.195)	Creamy Fruit Cup Snack (p.195)	Creamy Fruit Cup Snack (p.195)
DINNER	Marinated Tenderloin in Chipotle Sauce Dinner (p.133)	Marinated Tenderloin in Chipotle Sauce Dinner (p.133); Crustless Pumpkin Pie (p.231)	Marinated Tenderloin in Chipotle Sauce Dinner (p.133); Crustless Pumpkin Pie (p.231)	Marinated Tenderloin in Chipotle Sauce Dinner (p.133); Crustless Pumpkin Pie (p.231); 6 raw almonds
SNACK	Crab Bites Snacks (p.194)	1 sugar-free and fat-free popsicle	Buffalo Style Crackers (p.190)	½ pear
	39 grams fat / 1,228 calories	46 grams fat / 1,429 calories	53 grams fat / 1,643 calories	59.5 grams fat / 1,825 calories

Week 1 Day 4

	1,200 CALORIES	1,400 CALORIES	1,600 CALORIES	1,800 CALORIES
BREAKFAST	Buttermilk Pancakes with Sautéed Pears Breakfast (p.12); 1 tsp. light spread	Buttermilk Pancakes with Sautéed Pears Breakfast (p.12); 6 oz. reduced-fat (2%) milk	Buttermilk Pancakes with Sautéed Pears Breakfast (p.12); 1 oz. light cheddar cheese; ½ c. raspberries	Buttermilk Pancakes with Sautéed Pears Breakfast (p.12); 1 T. light spread; 4 T. light non-dairy whipped topping; ½ c. orange juice; 2 dried prunes
LUNCH	Roasted Pepper and Corn Soup (p. 34)	Roasted Pepper and Corn Soup (p.34); 1 c. light popcorn	Roasted Pepper and Corn Soup (p.34); 1 fat-free cracker; 1 tsp. soft spread	Roasted Pepper and Corn Soup (p.34) w/ 3 black olives; 2 c. light popcorn; 1 medium banana
SNACK	½ cup celery sticks w/ 1 T. fat-free Ranch dressing	½ c. celery sticks w/ 1 T. fat-free Ranch dressing	Garbanzo Nuts (p.188)	½ c. celery sticks w/ 1 T. fat-free Ranch dressing; 1 T. avocado
DINNER	Steamed Sea Bass with Creamy Buttermilk Coleslaw Dinner (p.159)	Steamed Sea Bass with Creamy Buttermilk Coleslaw Dinner (p.159); 2 tsp. light spread	Steamed Sea Bass with Creamy Buttermilk Coleslaw Dinner (p.159); Peach-Raspberry Tart (p.230)	Steamed Sea Bass with Creamy Buttermilk Coleslaw Dinner (p.159); Peach-Raspberry Tart (p.230)
SNACK	½ c. sugar-free flavored gelatin	½ c. sugar-free flavored gelatin; 4 oz. reduced-fat (2%) milk	Garden Vegetable Bruschetta Salad (p.204)	½ c. sugar-free flavored gelatin; ½ c. grapes; 3 walnuts
	39 grams fat / 1,215 calories	47.5 grams fat / 1,414 calories	53 grams fat / 1,646 calories	57 grams fat / 1,802 calories

Week 1 Day 5

	1,200 CALORIES	1,400 CALORIES	1,600 CALORIES	1,800 CALORIES
BREAKFAST	Scrunchy Berry Breakfast (p.9) w/ 2 T. light non-dairy whipped topping	Scrunchy Berry Breakfast (p.9) w/ 2 T. light non-dairy whipped topping	Scrunchy Berry Breakfast (p.9) w/ 2 T. non-fat non-dairy whipped topping; 1 oz. light cheddar cheese	Scrunchy Berry Breakfast (p.9); 1½ oz. light cheddar cheese; ¼ c. dried cranberries; 3 raw almonds
LUNCH	Roasted Red Pepper and Chicken Panini (p.68)	Roasted Red Pepper and Chicken Panini Lunch (p.68); 1 T. avocado	Roasted Red Pepper and Chicken Panini (p.68); 2 T. avocado; 1 medium apple	Roasted Red Pepper and Chicken Panini Lunch (p.68); 2 T. avocado; 1 c. salad greens w/ 1 T. fat-free Thousand Island dressing; 1 medium apple
SNACK	1 c. sliced cucumbers w/ 1 T. fat-free Thousand Island dressing	1 c. sliced cucumbers w/1 T. fat-free Thousand Island dressing	1 c. sliced cucumbers w/ 1 T. fat-free Thousand Island dressing	1 cup sliced cucumbers w/ 1 T. fat-free Thousand Island dressing
DINNER	Corn Cakes with Salmon and Dill Dinner (p.157)	Edamame Spread with Sesame Crisp (p.193); Corn Cakes with Salmon and Dill Dinner (p.157)	Edamame Spread with Sesame Crisp (p.193); Corn Cakes with Salmon and Dill Dinner (p.157); 5 large green olives	Edamame Spread with Sesame Crisp (p.193); Corn Cakes with Salmon and Dill Dinner (p.157); 3 black olives
SNACK	1 sugar-free and fat-free popsicle	Thai Shrimp Skewers (p.198)	1 sugar-free and fat-free popsicle; Thai Shrimp Skewers (p.198)	1 sugar-free and fat-free popsicle; Thai Shrimp Skewers (p.198)
	38 grams fat / 1,227 calories	45 grams fat / 1,418 calories	54 grams fat / 1,579 calories	58.5 grams fat / 1,794 calories

Week 1 Day 6

	1,200 CALORIES	1,400 CALORIES	1,600 CALORIES	1,800 CALORIES
BREAKFAST	Mixed Berry-Yogurt Smoothie Breakfast (p.4) w/ 2 T. light non-dairy whipped topping	Mixed Berry-Yogurt Smoothie Breakfast (p.4) w/ 2 T. light non-dairy whipped topping; ½ oz. light cheese	Mixed Berry-Yogurt Smoothie Breakfast (p.4) w/ 2 T. light non-dairy whipped topping; 6 oz. reduced-fat (2%) milk	Mixed Berry-Yogurt Smoothie Breakfast (p.4) w/ 2 T. light non-dairy whipped topping; 5 raw almonds; 3 prunes; 6 oz. reduced-fat (2%) milk
LUNCH	Simple Shrimp Paella (p.40)	Simple Shrimp Paella (p.40); 5 large green olives	Spicy Tuna Dip (p.192); Simple Shrimp Paella (p.40)	Spicy Tuna Dip (p.192); Simple Shrimp Paella (p.40); ½ oz. light cheddar cheese
SNACK	6 medium strawberries	16 oz. mineral water; ½ small orange	1 sugar-free and fat-free popsicle	16 oz mineral water; 2 orange slices; ½ c. grapes
DINNER	Southern Vegetarian Platter (p.182)	Black Bean Quesadillas (p.201); Southern Vegetarian Platter (p.182)	Black Bean Quesadillas (p.201); Southern Vegetarian Platter (p.182); 3 raw almonds	Black Bean Quesadillas (p.201); Southern Vegetarian Platter (p.182); 1 small orange; 6 raw almonds
SNACK	½ c. baby carrots with fat-free Ranch dressing	½ c. baby carrots w/ fat-free Ranch dressing	Maple-Glazed Popcorn (p.188)	½ c. sugar-free flavored gelatin;
	38 grams fat / 1,242 calories	47 grams fat / 1,441 calories	53 grams fat / 1,640 calories	57.5 grams fat / 1,832 calories

Week 1 Day 7

1,200 CALORIES	1,400 CALORIES	1,600 CALORIES	1,800 CALORIES
BREAKFAST Apple-Spice Muffins Breakfast (p.16); 1 tsp. light spread	Apple-Spice Muffins Breakfast (p.16); 1 c. low-fat fruit yogurt	Apple-Spice Muffins Breakfast (p.16); ½ c. low-fat fruit yogurt; 4 almonds	Apple-Spice Muffins Breakfast (p.16); 1 T. light spread; 6 oz. low-fat yogurt; ½ apple
LUNCH Grilled Chicken Burgers (p.70)	Grilled Chicken Burgers (p.70); 1 T. ⅓ less-fat cream cheese	Grilled Chicken Burgers (p.70); 1 T. light cream cheese; Lemon-Strawberry Sorbet (p.223)	Grilled Chicken Burgers Lunch (p.70); 1 ½ T. light mayonnaise; Lemon-Strawberry Sorbet (p.223)
SNACK ½ c. sugar-free flavored gelatin w/ 2 T. light non-dairy whipped topping	½ c. sugar-free flavored gelatin w/ 2 T. light non-dairy whipped topping	1 sugar-free, fat-free popsicle	½ c. sugar-free flavored gelatin w/ 4 T. light non-dairy whipped topping; 3 prunes
DINNER Ham and Steaks with Fruit Salsa Dinner (p.120)	Ham and Steaks with Fruit Salsa Dinner (p.120); 1 T. avocado	Ham and Steaks with Fruit Salsa Dinner (p.120); 4 walnuts and 1 c. greens w/ 1 T. fat-free Italian dressing	Ham and Steaks with Fruit Salsa Dinner (p.120); Peach-Raspberry Tart (p.230)
SNACK ½ c. mushrooms w/ 1 T. fat-free French dressing	½ c. mushrooms w/ 1 T. fat-free Ranch dressing	Chocolate-Banana Trifle (p.209)	½ c. mushrooms w/ 2 T. light Ranch dressing; 3 raw almonds
39 grams fat / 1,220 calories	47 grams fat / 1,405 calories	50 grams fat / 1,612 calories	59 grams fat / 1,814 calories

Week 2 Day 1

1,200 CALORIES	1,400 CALORIES	1,600 CALORIES	1,800 CALORIES
BREAKFAST Whole Grain Waffles with Berry Syrup (p.10)	Whole Grain Waffles with Berry Syrup (p.10); 4 oz. reduced-fat (2%) Milk	Whole Grain Waffles with Berry Syrup (p.10); 4 T. fat-free non-dairy whipped topping; 2 tsp. light spread; 1 small orange	Whole Grain Waffles with Berry Syrup (p.10); 2 T. light non-dairy whipped topping; 1 tsp. light spread; 1 medium banana
LUNCH Chesapeake Chicken Salad Lunch (p.50)	Edamame Spread with Sesame Crisp (p.193); Chesapeake Chicken Salad Lunch (p.50)	Chesapeake Chicken Salad Lunch (p.50); 1 T. avocado; Nutty Fruit Crisp (p.187)	Nutty Fruit Crisp (p. 187); Chesapeake Chicken Salad Lunch (p.50); 2 T. avocado; 3 dried figs
SNACK ½ cup sliced cucumber w/ 1 T. Ranch dressing	½ c. sliced cucumber w/ 1 T. fat-free Ranch dressing	½ cup sliced cucumber w/ 2 T. fat-free Ranch dressing; 3 walnuts	½ cup sliced cucumber w/ 2 T. fat-free Ranch dressing; 3 walnuts
DINNER Turkey Scaloppine Provencal Dinner (p.102)	Watermelon-Feta Crostini (p.194); Turkey Scaloppine Provencal Dinner (p.102)	Turkey Scaloppine Provencal Dinner (p.102); Watermelon-Feta Crostini (p.194)	Watermelon-Feta Crostini (p.194); Turkey Scaloppine Provencal Dinner (p.102); 3 black olives; ½ pear
SNACK Chocolate Pecan Roll (p.187)	½ c. sugar-free flavored gelatin w/ 4 T. light non-dairy whipped topping	3 raw almonds; 1 medium banana	½ c. carrot sticks
39 grams fat / 1,214 calories	46.5 grams fat / 1,417 calories	52 grams fat / 1,645 calories	58 grams fat / 1,816 calories

Week 2 Day 2

	1,200 CALORIES	1,400 CALORIES	1,600 CALORIES	1,800 CALORIES
BREAKFAST	1 c. bran flakes; 1 c. low-fat (1%) milk; ½ medium banana; 8 raw almonds	1 c. bran flakes; 1 c. low-fat (1%) milk; 8 raw walnuts; ½ oz. light mozzarella cheese; ½ cup grapes	1 c. bran flakes; 1 cup low-fat milk; 1 medium banana; 6 raw almonds and 2 T. sweet shredded coconut	1 c. bran flakes; 1 c. low-fat (1%) milk; 1 medium banana; 6 raw almonds; 2 T. sweet shredded coconut; 1 slice whole wheat bread; 2 tsp. light spread
LUNCH	Sausage and Pepper Sandwich (p.65)	Sausage and Pepper Sandwich (p.65)	Sausage and Pepper Sandwich (p.65)	Sausage and Pepper Sandwich (p.65); 1 medium orange; 1 c. salad greens w/ 1 T. fat-free Ranch dressing; 6 black olives
SNACK	16 oz. no-calorie flavored beverage	Trail Mix (p.190)	Trail Mix (p.190); 1 c. cup grapes	1 sugar-free and fat-free popsicle
DINNER	Orange Pork Roast Sauté Dinner (p.112)	Orange Pork Roast Sauté Dinner (p.112); 6 large green olives	Orange Pork Roast Sauté Dinner (p.112); Hot Apple Crunch (p.195); 2 T. light non-dairy whipped topping	Orange Pork Roast Sauté Dinner (p.112); Hot Apple Crunch (p.195); 4 T. light non-dairy whipped topping
SNACK	1 sugar-free and fat-free popsicle	1 sugar-free and fat-free popsicle	1 c. light popcorn	1 c. light popcorn; 1 small orange
	38 grams fat / 1,210 calories	47 grams fat / 1,403 calories	50 grams fat / 1,644 calories	57 grams fat / 1,820 calories

Week 2 Day 3

	1,200 CALORIES	1,400 CALORIES	1,600 CALORIES	1,800 CALORIES
BREAKFAST	Cheese Grits with Ham Breakfast (p.28)	Cheese Grits with Ham Breakfast (p.28); 1 T. ⅓-less-fat cream cheese	Cheese Grits with Ham Breakfast (p.28); 1 T. light cream cheese; 1 medium banana	Cheese Grits with Ham Breakfast (p.28); 2 T. light cream cheese; 1 pear; 1 walnut
LUNCH	Taco Salad (p.51)	Shiitake-Caramelized Onions Pizzas (p.202); Taco Salad (p.51)	Taco Salad Lunch (p.51); 1 T. avocado; 6 oz. cranberry juice	Shiitake-Caramelized Onions Pizzas (p.202); Taco Salad (p.51); 2 T. avocado; 6 oz. cranberry juice
SNACK	½ c. celery sticks w/ 1 T. fat-free Ranch dressing	½ c. celery sticks w/ 1 T. fat-free Ranch dressing	½ c. celery sticks w/ 1 T. fat-free Ranch dressing; 3 black olives	1 c. celery sticks w/ 1 T. fat-free Ranch dressing; 3 black olives
DINNER	Spring Vegetable Lasagna Dinner (p.166)	Spring Vegetable Lasagna Dinner (p.166); 1 T. avocado	Spring Vegetable Lasagna Dinner (p.166); Flourless Chocolate-Almond Cake (p.226)	Spring Vegetable Lasagna Dinner (p.166); Flourless Chocolate-Almond Cake (p.226); 6 T. light non-dairy whipped topping
SNACK	1 sugar-free and fat-free popsicle	Blueberry Polka Dot Pops (p.223)	1 sugar free and fat-free popsicle; 3 raw almonds	1 sugar-free and fat-free popsicle
	39 grams fat / 1,208 calories	47 grams fat / 1,443 calories	51 grams fat / 1,605 calories	59 grams fat / 1,805 calories

Week 2 Day 4

	1,200 CALORIES	1,400 CALORIES	1,600 CALORIES	1,800 CALORIES
BREAKFAST	Egg Muffin Sandwiches (p.22)	Egg Muffin Sandwiches (p.22); 2 T. avocado; 1 small orange	Egg Muffin Sandwiches (p.22); 3 T. avocado; 1 medium apple	Egg Muffin Sandwiches (p.22); 3 T. avocado; ½ medium apple; 1 c. low-fat fruit yogurt
LUNCH	Chunky Minestrone (p.36)	Chunky Minestrone (p.36); ½ c. reduced-fat (2%) Milk	Chunky Minestrone (p.36); ½ cup honey dew melon balls; Blueberry Polka Dot Pop (p.223)	Chunky Minestrone (p.36); Blueberry Polka Dot Pop (p.223); ½ c. honeydew melon cubes; 5 peanuts
SNACK	½ c. tomatoes chopped w/ lime juice and sprinkled w/ basil	½ c. tomatoes, chopped, w/ lime juice and sprinkled basil	½ cup tomatoes chopped w/ lime juice and sprinkled basil; 5 large green olives	½ c. tomatoes chopped w/ lime juice and sprinkled basil; ½ c. celery sticks; 5 large green olives
DINNER	Seared Cod with Steamed Vegetables Dinner (p.146)	Seared Cod with Steamed Vegetables Dinner (p.146); 6 raw almonds	Seared Cod with Steamed Vegetables Dinner (p.146); 1 slice non-fat bread and 1 T. light spread	Seared Cod with Steamed Vegetables Dinner (p.146); 1 slice light bread; 1 T. light spread; 5 peanuts; 1 small tangerine
SNACK	½ c. sugar-free flavored gelatin; 2 T. light non-dairy whipped topping	½ c. sugar-free flavored gelatin	½ c. sugar-free flavored gelatin	½ c. sugar-free flavored gelatin
	36 grams fat / 1,254 calories	46 grams fat / 1,433 calories	52 grams fat / 1,611 calories	60 grams fat / 1,830 calories

Week 2 Day 5

	1,200 CALORIES	1,400 CALORIES	1,600 CALORIES	1,800 CALORIES
BREAKFAST	Chilaquiles en Salsa Verde Breakfast (p.24); ½ c. reduced-fat (2%) milk	Chilaquiles en Salsa Verde Breakfast (p.24); 1 T. avocado; 1 kiwi	Chilaquiles en Salsa Verde Breakfast (p.24); 2 T. avocado; 2 black olives; 8 oz. orange juice	Chilaquiles en Salsa Verde Breakfast (p.24); 3 T. avocado; 3 black olives; 2 dried figs; 1 c. orange juice
LUNCH	Chopped Greek Salad with Steak Lunch (p.52)	Chopped Greek Salad with Steak Lunch (p.52); 1 T. light sour cream; ½ c. grapes	Chopped Greek Salad with Steak Lunch (p.52); 1 slice non-fat bread w/ 2 tsp. light spread; 1 small orange	Chopped Greek Salad with Steak Lunch (p.52); 2 slices light bread; 2 tsp. light spread; ¾ c. canned pears
SNACK	1 c. honeydew melon	Nutty Fruit Crisp (p.182)	4 oz. vanilla yogurt; 2 T. raisins	6 oz. low-fat fruit yogurt
DINNER	Easy Crab Cakes Dinner (p.142)	Easy Crab Cakes Dinner (p.142); 1 T. low-fat sour cream	Easy Crab Cakes Dinner (p.142); 1 T. low-fat sour cream; 3 raw almonds	Easy Crab Cakes Dinner (p.142); 2 T. low-fat sour cream; 3 walnuts; ½ canned peaches
SNACK	Mini Vegetable Croquettes (p.205)	Garbanzo Nuts (p.188)	Mini Vegetable Croquettes (p.205)	½ sugar-free fat-free flavored gelatin; 1 T. light non-dairy whipped topping
	38 grams fat / 1,219 calories	44 grams fat / 1,376 calories	52 grams fat / 1,605 calories	57 grams fat / 1,816 calories

Week 2 Day 6

	1,200 CALORIES	1,400 CALORIES	1,600 CALORIES	1,800 CALORIES
BREAKFAST	Watermelon-Strawberry Smoothies Breakfast (p.3)	Watermelon-Strawberry Smoothies Breakfast (p.3); ½ oz. light cheddar cheese	Watermelon-Strawberry Smoothies Breakfast (p.3); 4 T. light non-dairy whipped topping	Watermelon-Strawberry Smoothies Breakfast (p.3); 1½ oz. light cheddar cheese; ½ c. grapes
LUNCH	Tortellini Squash Soup (p.42)	Tortellini Squash Soup (p.42); 1 T. grated Parmesan cheese; 1 oz. light cheddar cheese	Tortellini Squash Soup (p.42); 2 T. grated Parmesan cheese; 1 medium banana	Tortellini Squash Soup (p.42); 1 T. grated Parmesan cheese; 1 medium banana; 5 peanuts
SNACK	½ c. sliced cucumbers w/ 1 T. fat-free Ranch dressing	½ c. sliced cucumbers w/ 1 T. fat-free Ranch dressing	½ cup sliced cucumbers w/ 2 T. fat-free Ranch dressing; 5 large green olives	½ c. sliced cucumbers w/ 2 T. fat-free Ranch dressing; 5 large green olives
DINNER	Linguine with Shrimp Scampi Dinner (p.160)	Garden Vegetable Bruschetta Salad (p.204); Linguine with Shrimp Scampi Dinner (p.160)	Linguine with Shrimp Scampi Dinner (p.160); Garden Vegetable Bruschetta Salad (p.204); 1 small orange	Garden Vegetable Bruschetta Salad (p.204); Linguine with Shrimp Scampi Dinner (p.160); 1 T. Parmesan cheese; 1 small orange
SNACK	½ cup mushrooms with 1 T. fat-free Ranch dressing	½ c. mushrooms w/ fat-free Ranch dressing	½ cup mushrooms with 1 T. fat-free Ranch dressing; 3 raw almonds	½ c. mushrooms w/ 1 T. fat-free Ranch dressing; ½ apple
	38 grams fat / 1,225 calories	47.5 grams fat / 1,391 grams fat	52 grams fat / 1,613 grams fat	60 grams fat / 1,805 grams fat

Week 2 Day 7

	1,200 CALORIES	1,400 CALORIES	1,600 CALORIES	1,800 CALORIES
BREAKFAST	Banana-Bran Muffins Breakfast (p.17)	Banana-Bran Muffins Breakfast (p.17); 1 T. light spread; ½ c. applesauce	Banana-Bran Muffins Breakfast (p.17); 1 T. light spread; ½ c. sweet applesauce	Banana-Bran Muffins Breakfast (p.17); 1 T. light spread; ½ cup sweet applesauce; 4 raw almonds
LUNCH	Cobb Salad with Salmon (p.57)	Cobb Salad with Salmon Lunch (p.57); 1 T. avocado; 1 small orange	Cobb Salad with Salmon Lunch (p.57); 2 T. avocado; ¾ c. grapes	Cobb Salad with Salmon Lunch (p.57); 2 T. avocado; Creamy Fruit Cup (p.195); ¾ c. grapes
SNACK	½ c. sugar-free flavored gelatin w/ 2 T. light non-dairy whipped topping	½ c. sugar-free flavored gelatin w/ 4 T. light non-dairy whipped topping	½ c. sugar-free flavored gelatin w/ 4 T. light non-dairy whipped topping	½ c. sugar-free flavored gelatin w/ 2 T. light non-dairy whipped topping
DINNER	Barbecued Chicken with Stir-Fried Vegetables Dinner (p.83)	Barbecued Chicken with Stir-Fried Vegetables Dinner (p.83)	Barbecued Chicken with Stir-Fried Vegetables Dinner (p.83); 1 oz. light cheddar cheese; 1 small orange	Barbecued Chicken with Stir-Fried Vegetables Dinner (p.83); 1 oz. light cheddar cheese; Peach-Raspberry Tart (p.230)
SNACK	Maple Glazed Popcorn (p.188)	Maple Glazed Popcorn (p.188)	Maple Glazed Popcorn (p.188)	Maple Glazed Popcorn (p.188)
	38 grams fat / 1,206 calories	46.5 grams fat / 1,436 calories	53 grams fat / 1,615 calories	60 grams fat / 1,788 calories

Week 3 Day 1

	1,200 CALORIES	1,400 CALORIES	1,600 CALORIES	1,800 CALORIES
BREAKFAST	Ricotta Pancakes with Dried Fruit Sauce (p.11)	Ricotta Pancakes with Dried Fruit Sauce (p.11)	Ricotta Pancakes with Dried Fruit Sauce (p.11); 3 T. light non-dairy whipped topping	Ricotta Pancakes with Dried Fruit Sauce (p.11); 4 T. non-dairy whipped topping; 3 almonds; ½ c. low-fat fruit yogurt
LUNCH	Simple Shrimp Paella (p.40)	Simple Shrimp Paella (p.40); ½ T. light spread	Stuffed Mushrooms (p.200); Simple Shrimp Paella (p.40)	Stuffed Mushrooms (p.200); Simple Shrimp Paella (p.40)
SNACK	16 oz. mineral water w/ ¼ c. sliced oranges	16 oz. mineral water w/ ¼ c. sliced oranges	16 oz. mineral water w/ ¼ c. sliced oranges	16 oz. mineral water; ¼ c. sliced oranges; Trail Mix (p. 190)
DINNER	Turkey and Sweet Potato Stew (p.106)	Turkey and Sweet Potato Stew (p.106); Chocolate-Banana Trifle (p.209); 2 T. light non-dairy whipped topping	Turkey and Sweet Potato Stew Dinner (p.106); Chocolate-Banana Trifle (p.209); 2 T. light non-dairy whipped topping	Turkey and Sweet Potato Stew Dinner (p.106); Chocolate-Banana Trifle (p.209)
SNACK	1 sugar-free, fat-free popsicle	1 sugar-free, fat-free popsicle	Peach-Raspberry Tart (p.230)	Peach-Raspberry Tart (p.230)
	38 grams fat / 1,225 calories	44.5 grams fat / 1,382 calories	53 grams fat / 1,650 calories	58 grams fat / 1,866 calories

Week 3 Day 2

	1,200 CALORIES	1,400 CALORIES	1,600 CALORIES	1,800 CALORIES
BREAKFAST	Soul Frittata Breakfast (p.29)	Soul Frittata Breakfast (p.29); 4 oz. reduced-fat (2%) milk; ½ small orange	Soul Frittata Breakfast (p.29); 2 T. light sour cream; 1 c. grapes; 3 walnuts	Soul Frittata Breakfast (p.29); 2 T. light sour cream; 1½ c. grapes; 6 walnuts
LUNCH	Chicken and White Bean Chili Lunch (p.35)	Chicken and White Bean Chili Lunch (p.35); 6 almonds	Chicken and White Bean Chili Lunch (p.35); Fruit Salad with Frozen Yogurt (p.222)	Chicken and White Bean Chili Lunch (p.35); Fruit Salad with Frozen Yogurt (p.222)
SNACK	½ c. sugar-free flavored gelatin	½ c. sugar-free flavored gelatin	½ c. sugar-free flavored gelatin; 4 T. light non-dairy whipped topping	½ c. sugar-free flavored gelatin; 4 T. light non-dairy whipped topping
DINNER	Hearty Manhattan Clam Chowder Dinner (p.144)	Hearty Manhattan Clam Chowder Dinner (p.144); Stuffed Mushrooms (p.200); 1 T. avocado	Stuffed Mushrooms (p.200); Hearty Manhattan Clam Chowder Dinner (p.144)	Black Bean Quesadillas (p.201); Hearty Manhattan Clam Chowder Dinner (p.144); 2 T. avocado; 1 kiwi
SNACK	½ c. jicama sticks w/ 1 tsp. fresh lemon juice and 5 green olives	½ c. jicama sticks w/ 1 tsp. fresh lemon juice	½ c. jicama sticks w/ 1 tsp. fresh lemon juice; 5 green olives	½ c. jicama sticks w/ 1 tsp. fresh lemon juice; 5 green olives
	39 grams fat / 1,207 calories	48.5 grams fat / 1,429 calories	53 grams fat / 1,639.5 calories	60 grams fat / 1,823 calories

Week 3 Day 3

	1,200 CALORIES	1,400 CALORIES	1,600 CALORIES	1,800 CALORIES
BREAKFAST	Apple-Cinnamon Oatmeal (p.5)	Apple-Cinnamon Oatmeal Breakfast (p.5); ½ c. low-fat fruit yogurt	Apple-Cinnamon Oatmeal Breakfast (p.5); 3 raw almonds; ½ large banana	Apple-Cinnamon Oatmeal (p.5); 6 raw almonds; 1 large banana
LUNCH	Gazpacho Salad with Goat Cheese (p.60)	Gazpacho Salad with Goat Cheese (p.60)	Gazpacho Salad with Goat Cheese (p.60); Crustless Pumpkin Pie (p.231)	Gazpacho Salad with Goat Cheese (p.60); Crustless Pumpkin Pie (p.231)
SNACK	½ c. celery sticks w/ 1 T. fat-free Ranch dressing	½ c. celery sticks w/ 1 T. fat-free Ranch dressing	½ c. celery sticks w/ 1 T. fat-free Ranch dressing	Garden Vegetable Bruschetta Salad (p.204)
DINNER	Blackberry Pork Tenderloin Dinner (p.108)	Edamame Spread with Sesame Crisp (p.193); Blackberry Pork Tenderloin Dinner (p.108)	Edamame Spread with Sesame Crisp (p.193); Blackberry Pork Tenderloin Dinner (p.108); ½ c. honeydew melon	Edamame Spread with Sesame Crisp (p.193); Blackberry Pork Tenderloin Dinner (p.108); ½ c. honeydew; 5 green olives
SNACK	1 sugar-free, fat-free popsicle	Mini Vegetable Croquettes (p.205)	Mini Vegetable Croquettes (p.205); 1 T. light cream cheese	Mini Vegetable Croquettes (p.205); 1 T. light cream cheese
	40 grams fat / 1,230 calories	46.5 grams fat / 1,439 calories	51 grams fat / 1,646 calories	58.5 grams fat / 1,793 calories

Week 3 Day 4

	1,200 CALORIES	1,400 CALORIES	1,600 CALORIES	1,800 CALORIES
BREAKFAST	Scrambled Egg Cups Breakfast (p.21)	Scrambled Egg Cups Breakfast (p.21); 4 oz. reduced-fat (2%) milk	Scrambled Egg Cups Breakfast (p.21) 2 T. avocado; ¾ c. blueberries	Scrambled Egg Cups Breakfast (p.21) 2 T. avocado; 4 T. light non-dairy whipped topping; 1½ c. blueberries
LUNCH	Chunky Minestrone (p.36)	Chunky Minestrone (p.36); 2 T. light sour cream	Chunky Minestrone (p.36); 2 T. light sour cream	Chunky Minestrone (p.36); 2 T. light sour cream
SNACK	½ c. cucumber slices w/ lemon juice	½ c. coleslaw chopped w/ 1 T. fat-free, sugar-free plain yogurt	½ c. coleslaw chopped w/ 1 T. fat-free and sugar-free plain yogurt	Hot Apple Crunch (p.195)
DINNER	Barbecued Salmon with Collards, Okra, and Tomato Dinner (p.154)	Barbecued Salmon with Collards, Okra, and Tomato Dinner (p.154); 1 ½ c. greens w/ 1 T. fat-free Italian dressing	Barbecued Salmon with Collards, Okra, and Tomato Dinner (p.154); Butterscotch Fondue (p.211)	Barbecued Salmon with Collards, Okra, and Tomato Dinner (p.154); Butterscotch Fondue (p.211); 2 walnuts
SNACK	½ c. sugar-free flavored gelatin w/ 2 T. light non-dairy whipped topping	½ cup sugar-free flavored gelatin w/ 2 T. light non-dairy whipped topping; ½ c. canned light fruit cocktail	½ c. sugar free flavored gelatin w/ 6 T. light non-dairy whipped topping; ½ c. light fruit cocktail	Tiramisu (p.212); ½ c. light fruit cocktail
	38 grams fat / 1,215 calories	46 grams fat / 1,435 calories	50 grams fat / 1,612 calories	57.5 grams fat / 1,822 calories

Week 3 Day 5

	1,200 CALORIES	1,400 CALORIES	1,600 CALORIES	1,800 CALORIES
BREAKFAST	Fruit-Topped Breakfast Pizza Breakfast (p.20)	Fruit-Topped Breakfast Pizza Breakfast (p.20); 2 walnuts	Fruit-Topped Breakfast Pizza Breakfast (p.20); 3 T. light cream cheese; ½ pear	Fruit-Topped Breakfast Pizza Breakfast (p.20); 2 T. light cream cheese; 1 pear; 6 almonds
LUNCH	Canadian BLTs (p.66)	Canadian BLTs (p.66); ½ c. low-fat fruit yogurt	Canadian BLTs (p.66); 1 T. avocado; ½ c. low-fat fruit yogurt	Canadian BLTs (p.66); 2 T. avocado; 1 c. low-fat fruit yogurt
SNACK	16 oz. mineral water w/ 2 T. berries	16 oz. mineral water w/ 2 T. berries	16 oz. mineral water w/ 2 T. berries; 1 medium banana	16 oz. mineral water; 2 T. berries; 1 medium banana; 3 almonds
DINNER	White Bean and Escarole Ragout (p.178)	White Bean and Escarole Ragout (p.178); 1 T. grated Parmesan cheese	White Bean and Escarole Ragout (p.178); 1 T. grated Parmesan cheese	White Bean and Escarole Ragout Dinner (p.178); 1 T. grated Parmesan Cheese
SNACK	1½ cups light popcorn	Flourless Chocolate-Almond Cake (p.226)	2 c. light popcorn	3 c. light popcorn
	38 grams fat / 1,199 calories	45.5 grams fat / 1,427 calories	51 grams fat / 1,625 calories	59.5 grams fat / 1,810 calories

Week 3 Day 6

	1,200 CALORIES	1,400 CALORIES	1,600 CALORIES	1,800 CALORIES
BREAKFAST	1 large slice multi-grain bread; 2 T. light cream cheese; 2 T. avocado; ½ c. peach slices	1 medium bagel; 4 T. light cream cheese; ½ c. vanilla yogurt	1 medium bagel; 4 T. light cream cheese; 2 T. avocado; 1 c. light canned peaches	1 medium whole wheat bagel; 4 T. light cream cheese; 3 T. avocado; ¾ c. light canned peaches
LUNCH	Winter Salad Delight (p.54)	Winter Salad Delight (p.54); 3 large green olives	Winter Salad Delight (p.54); 1 c. grapes; 6 raw almonds	Winter Salad Delight (p.54); 1 c. grapes; 9 raw almonds
SNACK	½ c. sliced cucumbers w/ 1 T. fat-free Ranch dressing	½ c. sliced cucumbers w/ 2 T. fat-free Ranch dressing	½ cup sliced cucumbers w/ 1 T. fat-free Ranch dressing; 5 large green olives	Spicy Tuna Dip (p.192);
DINNER	Chicken with Snap Peas (p.86)	Chicken with Snap Peas (p.86)	Chicken with Snap Peas (p.86)	Chicken with Snap Peas Dinner (p.86); 5 green olives
SNACK	1 sugar-free, fat-free popsicle	½ cup sugar-free gelatin w/ 2 T. light non-dairy whipped topping	Garbanzo Nuts (p.188)	Garbanzo Nuts (p.188)
	39.5 grams fat / 1,245 calories	45.5 grams fat / 1,411 calories	53 grams fat / 1,645 calories	60 grams fat / 1,785 calories

Week 3 Day 7

	1,200 CALORIES	1,400 CALORIES	1,600 CALORIES	1,800 CALORIES
BREAKFAST	Raspberry-Sour Cream Muffins (p.15)	Raspberry-Sour Cream Muffins (p.15); 2 T. light non-dairy whipped topping	Raspberry-Sour Cream Muffins (p.15); 1 T. light spread; 1 medium banana	Raspberry-Sour Cream Muffins (p.15); 1 T. light spread; 1 medium banana
LUNCH	Herbed Tuna and White Bean Salad (p.56)	Herbed Tuna and White Bean Salad (p.56); 1 small orange	Herbed Tuna and White Bean Salad (p.56); Lemon Cheesecake Parfait (p.214)	Herbed Tuna and White Bean Salad (p.56); Lemon Cheesecake Parfait (p.214); 2 walnuts
SNACK	½ c. sugar-free flavored gelatin w/ 2 T. light non-dairy whipped topping	½ c. sugar-free flavored gelatin	½ c. sugar-free flavored gelatin	Shiitake-Caramelized Onion Pizzas (p.202)
DINNER	Peppered Beef Tenderloin Dinner (p.122)	Peppered Beef Tenderloin Dinner (p.122); Pears with Maple Crème (p.216)	Peppered Beef Tenderloin Dinner (p.122); Pears with Maple Crème (p.216)	Peppered Beef Tenderloin Dinner (p.122); Pears with Maple Crème (p.216); 5 almonds
SNACK	1 c. strawberries	Summer Roasted Fruit Kabobs (p.216) w/ 2 T. light non-dairy whipped topping	Summer Roasted Fruit Kabobs (p.216)	Summer Roasted Fruit Kabobs (p.216); 2 T. light non-dairy whipped topping
	38 grams fat / 1,204 calories	44.5 grams fat / 1,426 calories	50 grams fat / 1,628 calories	58 grams fat / 1,787 calories

index

Numbers in **boldface** indicate photo pages for finished dishes.

about the authors

Kathleen Daelemans

Chef Kathleen's recipes have been showcased in respected food and wine journals including *Bon Appetit*, *Wine Spectator*, *Gourmet*, *Food & Wine*, and *Eating Well*. No stranger to television, Chef Kathleen wrote and hosted a weekly Food Network show, *Cooking Thin with Kathleen Daelemans*, and her insights, recipes, and kitchen tricks and tips continue to enrich and entertain audiences through her regular television appearances.

When it comes to healthy cooking and eating, Ms. Daelemans is "her own best advertisement," having lost 75 pounds when creating a new regional cuisine for one of the world's most luxurious five-star resort and spas, The Grand Wailea, in Maui, Hawaii. Whether on TV, on the national lecture circuit, or as a spokesperson on national media satellite campaigns, she continues to promote a healthy lifestyle every day of the year while still enjoying great food. Ms. Daelemans is the author of *Cooking Thin and Getting Thin and Loving Food*.

Sylvia Meléndez-Klinger, M.S., R.D., L.D., C.P.T

An expert in cross-cultural cuisine as it relates to nutrition and health, Sylvia Meléndez-Klinger leverages tasteful Latin cuisine with a healthy lifestyle. Ms. Klinger is a culinary consultant to food and beverage companies such as General Mills, The Coca-Cola Company, and Hormel. A registered dietitian and certified personal trainer, Ms. Klinger is founder of Hispanic Food Communications, a food communications and culinary consulting company.

Ms. Klinger is a member of the American Dietetic Association and Latino Hispanic American Dietetic Association, as well as Dietitians in Business & Communications, and Food and Culinary Professionals Practice Groups. She is an active member of the Chicago and Illinois Dietetic Associations and a member of the Grain Foods Foundation Advisory Board.

Lindsey Williams

Lindsey Williams, the grandson of Harlem's queen of soul food, Sylvia Woods, is a former record executive and now the owner of Neo Soul Events and Catering, a complete event planning and catering company.

Mr. Williams grew up in the kitchen of his grandmother's legendary restaurant, where he learned the art of authentic soul food cooking. But he was also always overweight, and when he tipped the scales at 400 pounds, he knew he had to make some drastic changes. Mr. Williams completely changed his lifestyle and his diet, lost more than half his weight, and eventually created his own brand of healthy soul food cooking.

Lindsey Williams is the author of *Neo Soul: Taking Soul Food to a Whole 'Nutha' Level*, a cookbook that offers soul food favorites with a healthy twist.